Praise for *Embrace Your Best Self*

Embrace Your Best Self: Fabulous and Healthy After 50 *is a refreshing reminder that life is not over after fifty; on the contrary, a new season of life is just beginning! This hands-on guide to a stronger, healthier lifestyle is filled with practical advice to move the silver-haired generation into the future with courage and optimism.*

It is a welcome addition to my cache of inspirational reserves that I shall indulge in time and time again.

Shirley A. Turner, Ph.D.
English Language Arts (ELA) Instructional Coach, In Touch Consulting LLC

Dr. McLymont takes us on a journey to reclaim our lives with joy, grace, and wisdom. Her uplifting writing and charming anecdotes inspire us to take positive steps toward nourishing the body, mind, and spirit. No matter your age, this book will give you the tools you need to embrace your best self.

Roseanne Schnoll, PhD, RD, CDN
Associate Professor / Director, Dietetic Internship, Brooklyn College

Dr. McLymont has captured and synthesized all of the key aspects of healthy living in one place. She provides a thoughtful and well researched book that is a must read for anybody interested in adopting a healthy lifestyle.

Mark Schattner, MD, AGAF, FASGE
Chief, Gastroenterology, Hepatology and Nutrition Service, MSK Professor of Clinical Medicine, Weil Cornell College of Medicine

The first time I met Dr. Veronica I thought she was my colleague's sister. Instead I quickly learned she was her mother! Dr. Veronica is the amazing epitome of timeless beauty and grace. She is the ultimate expression of the mind, body, spirit connection we all aspire to. I have been honored to be on the receiving end of her conversations and counsel around health, beauty, and aging. As a woman transitioning into another stage of my life, I'm glad to have this book as a ready reference and source of positive encouragement on my journey.

Carla Moore
VP, Sales Strategy and Education, HBO

I have had the great fortune to witness Veronica's positivity, pride, and presence as they have propelled her successful career and inspired others to be their best! She meets life's challenges with confidence and enthusiasm! Thanks for sharing your unique gifts in this book and being a role model for women of all ages!

Sharon Cox, LD, RD
Owner/Co-Founder Cox Duncan Network, LLC

Embrace
Your
Best Self

Veronica McLymont, PhD

Embrace *Your* Best Self

FABULOUS & HEALTHY AFTER

50

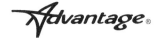

Published by Advantage, Charleston, South Carolina.
Member of Advantage Media Group.

ADVANTAGE is a registered trademark, and the Advantage colophon is a trademark of Advantage Media Group, Inc.

Printed in the United States of America.

10 9 8 7 6 5 4 3 2 1

ISBN: 978-1-59932-831-7
LCCN: 2017964415

Book design by Megan Elger.

This publication is designed to provide accurate and authoritative information in regard to the subject matter covered. It is sold with the understanding that the publisher is not engaged in rendering legal, accounting, or other professional services. If legal advice or other expert assistance is required, the services of a competent professional person should be sought.

Advantage Media Group is proud to be a part of the Tree Neutral® program. Tree Neutral offsets the number of trees consumed in the production and printing of this book by taking proactive steps such as planting trees in direct proportion to the number of trees used to print books. To learn more about Tree Neutral, please visit **www.treeneutral.com**.

Advantage Media Group is a publisher of business, self-improvement, and professional development books and online learning. We help entrepreneurs, business leaders, and professionals share their Stories, Passion, and Knowledge to help others Learn & Grow. Do you have a manuscript or book idea that you would like us to consider for publishing? Please visit **advantagefamily.com** or call **1.866.775.1696**.

To all the women over fifty who have influenced me to continuously better myself and didn't even know it. I thank you.

Table of Contents

part three: your best spirit

about the author

Dr. Veronica McLymont holds a PhD in organizational leadership from the University of Maryland Eastern Shore, an MS in nutrition from Hunter College, and a BS in foods and nutrition from Brooklyn College. She is a registered and certified dietitian-nutritionist (RDN, CDN) and a certified professional life coach.

Dr. McLymont was voted a "Trendsetter" by the American Society for Healthcare Food Service Administrators. She was also recognized as one of the twenty-five "Most Influential Black Women in Business" by the *Network Journal*. She received the Award for Excellence in Management Practice from the Academy of Nutrition and Dietetics, in addition to the Exemplary Leadership Award from the Association for Healthcare Foodservice. She was named one of the Top Women in Metro New York Foodservice and Hospitality by *Total Foodservice Magazine*.

Dr. McLymont is the author of the chapter "Nutrition Care of the Cancer Patient" in *Cancer Rehabilitation: Principles and Practice,* a cancer rehabilitation textbook. She has also *coauthored a chapter* in the textbook, *Research: Successful Approaches*, as well as contributing to several research papers. She has given numerous lectures on nutrition and leadership-related topics and is viewed as an industry resource.

Dr. McLymont has served as president and board member for several professional organizations. She lives and works in the health care industry in New York City.

foreword

Growing older has many advantages, one of which is the opportunity to reassess the people in your life and whether or not they bring you joy and add value to your life. I'm happy to say that Veronica McLymont will always make the list.

Veronica is the sage advice of your grandmother. She is the older sister with the wisdom needed in every situation you'll encounter because she's experienced it all.

Veronica, what took you so long?! We've been waiting! We needed your inspiration, your wit, your humility, and your courage to share your vast knowledge and real life experiences we could relate to at any age.

Thanks for standing up to empower women over fifty to believe they're *still* fabulous and *still* have so much more of life to live, love, and explore!

Veronica obviously practices what she puts in print. And you can now put her on your list of valuable people. She's going to change your life!

Brenda Blackmon
Multi-Emmy Award Winning TV Journalist

acknowledgment

This book is in acknowledgment of my daughter Antoinette Miller. She is my proudest accomplishment and has always kept me grounded. Antoinette, you were born ready. Keep walking with confidence, class, consistency, and a whole lotta courage!

I love you.
Mom

introduction

Aging—Why Not Embrace Your Best?

It was a warm summer day in New York City as I stood eagerly waiting for my longtime college friend, Marsha, to meet me in Central Park for a picnic.

I was excited at the thought of seeing Marsha since we hadn't seen each other in over a decade. Marsha and I had remained friends after college, even though she moved from the East Coast to California right after graduation.

When she arrived at the park, we could have spotted each other from a mile away. "Marsha!" "Veronica!" We exclaimed at the same time as we hugged each other. We looked each other up and down, and I realized that we both looked great, yet slightly different— changes in appearance can be very apparent when you haven't seen someone for a very long time.

Just like in our college days we chatted, giggled like schoolgirls, and raved about our respective lives. We went from one topic to the next, delving into our careers, our marriages, and of course, our children. In a strange way, after all those years, it was really thrilling to see my friend and reconnect.

It was then that I blurted, "Can you believe we're over fifty?"

She quickly quipped, "So what if we are over fifty? I'm embracing it!" She spoke of aging as if it was a great accomplishment, a special "badge" of sorts to be proudly displayed for the world to see what it meant to live life fully well into her fifties.

Her words took me by complete surprise. Instead of a typical reply like, "Oh, yes, we're getting older," or, "We're not getting any younger," my friend had a completely different outlook. In fact, after I thought about it for a second, I realized that Marsha's response made a lot of sense, and it reassured me. Because she was right—we are meant to embrace our age, even if we are over fifty.

For me, embracing my age meant feeling confident in my skin. It meant, after years spent raising my daughter and succeeding in my career, that, *I'm the best I've ever been.* And now that I've hit my stride in life, I don't want to stop. I want to keep going. *I want to embrace my age, but I want to be fabulous and healthy beyond fifty,* I thought. *Why not embrace it then?*

> **Now that I've hit my stride in life, I don't want to stop. I want to keep going.**

Yet, Marsha's outlook goes against popular culture. Sure, aging is perfectly natural, but society regards it as something to shun, cover up, or fix altogether. We see it every day—we are confronted with an overwhelming number of anti-aging products in stores, TV ads, and magazine spreads that focus on looking youthful.

Meanwhile, in comparison, there are far fewer portrayals of women over fifty in the media—women who are accomplished, strong, and confident. You get the impression that older women with these attributes recede into the background as their youth wanes. But there's much more to our lives than superficial youthful appearance.

To challenge society's views about aging, we sometimes brush them off by saying, "Age is just a number," "Age is just a state of mind," or, "Fifty is the new thirty." But few of us—including me before that moment in Central Park with Marsha—understand that our years bring an unfathomable depth of fabulousness that we shouldn't allow to go to waste.

"Embrace your best" isn't just another cliché. *Embrace your best* means understanding that your best—your experiences and your lifetime of achievements, like raising a family or career successes—is a fountain of youth of sorts, one that you can tap into, enjoy, and share. *Embrace your best* means that, in this moment, you are stronger, wiser, and more accomplished than you've ever been. So, instead of looking back, look at who you are today. Life after fifty becomes a new chapter, a new adventure on which to embark. It becomes very liberating to embrace your best.

That's why I wrote this book: *Embrace Your Best Self: Fabulous and Healthy Beyond Fifty*. It's for women who look in the mirror and fret over graying strands of hair. It's for women who experience emptiness after their children move out of the house. It's for women who vow to devote more time to honoring their authentic selves. In this book, I will pass on knowledge I've learned over the years about aging, especially past fifty. The stories I share will help you on your journey to age gracefully and stay fabulous and healthy.

I believe that when you adopt a positive mindset, take better care of your health, and nurture your spirit, you can become the best version of yourself. So when the topic of age arises today, I gladly repeat the wise words of my friend Marsha: "*Embrace it!*" I am the best I've ever been.

To show you how to accomplish your best, I've divided this book into three parts.

- *Part One: Your Best Mind* explains why now is the time to take care of yourself, how to share yourself with others, what kind of opportunities you'll discover when you break out of your comfort zone, and why slowing your pace can be one of the best things you can do for yourself.

- *Part Two: Your Best Body* is about a healthier, fabulous you, and shares ideas for beauty beyond fifty, nutrition for life, and exercises for your mind, body, and overall health.

- *Part Three: Your Best Spirit* encourages you to give thanks every day. It offers ideas for affirming your best self to keep tough times from lingering and to let you know that better days are ahead. At the end of each chapter, you'll find takeaways to help you embrace your best as well as exercises to help you practice concepts from the chapter. They will show you that you have the resources to stay fabulous and healthy while you have the time of your life.

That's right—when you embrace aging, don't be surprised when people tell you that you don't look your age.

Be Fabulous, Live Healthy

If you're going through a transition and feel like you're just getting older, then in the pages ahead you'll find ways to rejuvenate, ways to stay physically and socially active, ways to feel connected, as well as new things you can explore and enjoy. In essence, you'll find a graceful aging guide to transform your changing life to a "changed you."

Throughout my career as a registered dietitian-nutritionist, I have been responsible for managing staff in large medical centers. But in my early thirties, while I was a practicing dietitian working directly with patients, it was striking to see people—many of them women—battling a host of debilitating illnesses well before they reached middle age. I saw obesity, diabetes, high blood pressure, cancer, and heart disease prevent them from living full, productive lives. In many cases, better nutrition could have prevented their downward spiral, staving off the physical changes associated with aging. But good nutrition is just one piece of what it takes to be healthy in mind, body, and spirit.

> **In the pages ahead you'll find a graceful aging guide to transform your changing life to a "changed you."**

Those past experiences in my professional role have taught me plenty—I've learned to be optimistic and receptive to change, to be assertive, to respond to the needs of others, to show empathy, to have self-confidence, to be resilient, and to remain emotionally stable. Today I use these attributes to build relationships and empower others.

Over time, sharing my insights with others has gradually evolved into mentorships. I've mentored others, including veterans, and provided them with professional guidance. Eventually, I was inspired to become a life coach. I realized that, as a coach, I would have to be certified, authentic, approachable, nonjudgmental, and a very good listener. Above all, I had to have an open mind. Coaching and mentoring are different in how they are applied, but both give me a deeper understanding of the issues that others, especially aging women, face today.

The chapters ahead are designed to encourage you to overcome reservations about aging, embrace your best, and be fabulous and healthy beyond fifty.

Be Fabulous: Live with the Three Ps

Living with the three Ps—*positivity, pride,* and *presence*—is the foundation for an exciting next chapter in your life.

Positivity

Living with *positivity* is about being upbeat and choosing to live in an environment that pleases you. It's having an optimistic viewpoint even when negative situations arise. It's getting up, dressing, and showing up no matter how you feel. It's finding the humor in things. It's avoiding being inundated with the "noise" and negative information. When you focus on the positive, it overshadows the negative. It's going after your dreams, and not letting your fears prevent you from living your dreams. It's thinking about your purpose in life— what has it been up to this point? Research shows that having a sense of purpose in life could add years to your life.[1] What positive things can you do to improve the world? Think about what makes you feel happy and fulfilled. What will keep you in balance—physically, mentally, and spiritually—in the years ahead and give you a bright new perspective on being over fifty?

---

1   Andrew Steptoe, Angus Deacon, and Arthur Stone, "Subjective wellbeing, health, and ageing," *The Lancet* 385, no. 9968 (February 2015): 640-648.

Pride

Living with *pride* is about shaking off the old double standard and not worrying about your age. Pride in yourself after fifty means you can pursue your passions, meet people, make new friends, and embrace the best years of your life. It doesn't mean retiring from life. Instead, it's ushering in life and knowing the value of celebrating it. It's being passionate about looking forward to the good that lies ahead, and realizing how much more there is. Pride is the freeing feeling that menopause is behind you and knowing that you sizzle. Enjoy your sensuality and sexuality. You have wisdom and experience to your credit. You don't look old, feel old, or act old. You believe in yourself and are proud of it. Pride is knowing that the sky is the limit, and that you can thrive anywhere. As you start to find new ways to rejuvenate, be ready to adapt and proudly embrace the changes that come after fifty. It means having greater self-trust and knowing who you are. So take pride in looking good and feeling good about your age.

Presence

Living with *presence* means you exude charm, confidence, boldness, and passion. Nothing can take the place of presence. It's a reflection of the energy you put out. Presence draws people to you. Your good qualities get noticed when you have presence. What you say, and how you say it, matters. Presence is being fierce. It's walking into a room and owning it. It makes people ask, "Who was that woman?" Presence is being mindful. When you're mindful, you're taking stock of things around you and in your life. Presence is about "more." When you wake up in the morning, you're more mindful of how you want your day to go. You become the strongest, most passionate version of yourself when you have presence.

part one

Your Best Mind

chapter one

You Have Arrived!

Sabrina, age fifty-one, was a registered nurse who's spent her life taking care of others, both at work and at home. When she wasn't busy raising the kids and running her household, she was at the hospital managing an inpatient unit of critically ill patients and leading a large team of nurses. But, even after a busy twelve-hour shift, and still dressed in hospital scrubs, it was clear she was an incredibly fabulous woman—but I don't think she ever paused to think of herself in that light.

One day, passing each other in the hall, Sabrina and I stopped and chatted for a while about our daughters, who were then both in college, and our lives without them.

"Where did the years go?" she asked.

If you've reached middle age, you've most likely asked yourself this question. Looking back, I'm sure you feel that the years passed by rather quickly. Admittedly, like Sabrina, I felt that those demanding years of working and raising my daughter flew by with me barely realizing it.

The funny thing is, time doesn't just pass by—it adds up. Aging is like weight gain that creeps up on you without you noticing. Then that fateful day comes when your jeans don't fit and the face in the mirror is nearly unrecognizable, and you wonder, "Is that me?"

But when it comes to aging, we have much more to show for our years than an older face in the mirror and aching joints. We are more than the sum of our wrinkles and pains.

With age comes a great deal of wisdom and experience that we can put to good use. It starts with taking care of *ourselves*.

This became clear working in healthcare and being surrounded by caregivers on a daily basis. I saw the toll that caring for *others* can take. In many cases, caregivers put others first at the cost of their own self-care. We should all stop and ask, "Who's caring for the caregiver?"

Have you made sacrifices for others? Now's the time to make sacrifices for yourself. Have you "let yourself go"? Now's the time to take charge of your health. Were you too busy with your career and raising a family? Now's the time to slow down and focus on things you really want to do.

Whether it's attending to family, friends, or your company and its customers, chances are you too have been putting others first. Whatever form your caregiving takes, there comes a time when you must find ways to replenish what's been depleted. Without taking care of yourself, you won't be resilient enough to be there for others.

If you're asking, "Why now?" Well, if not now, when? You've earned the right to put yourself first. If your kids are grown, and you no longer work, you are likely to have fewer responsibilities. This is the perfect time to make yourself a priority. No more running to day care, no more shuttling kids to after-school activities. No more rushing from work, juggling to make evening classes or cramming for exams.

That feeling of finally being free to take care of yourself and to do more of what you want is liberating—but it can also be a bit scary. Some people call it the "empty nest syndrome." It sometimes shows up as a "midlife crisis," or being "over the hill." These worries stem from the same notion that our best years are behind us and that we're approaching *the end*. It's like a movie is over, the credits are rolling on the screen, the audience is exiting the theater, and there you are alone in your seat as the house lights come on and the usher sweeps up the popcorn.

Rather than seeing this as the *end,* think of this time as the *beginning of your new chapter*. Your new chapter must therefore take two approaches: being **fabulous** and being **healthy**. If you're fabulous and healthy, it shows that you are looking forward and not backward, taking care of yourself, getting over your midlife and empty nest worries, and embracing your best.

You're Already Fabulous

Going back to Sabrina's story, I told her the same thing I'm saying to you now: "Look at you. You are fabulous and accomplished. At this age, it is possible that stuff happened—and the everyday stops and restarts have zapped your self-confidence. You may be reminiscing, looking back, nostalgic for youth. Now's the time to take stock."

If you're like Sabrina, maybe the very idea of being fabulous after fifty never crossed your mind. But somewhere in your travels you've seen *her*. When you see *her*, that oh-so-put-together woman of a certain age—over fifty or sixty but looking like forty and flaunting it like twenty—you can't help but wonder, *how does she do it?*

Maybe *she* is a friend who looks so good that you ask, "You look great! What are you taking?" Or better yet, "Did you have something done?" *She* knows she's fabulous. She's tapped into her experience and owns it. She's proud of her achievements in her personal and professional life. She knows she has to take good care of herself. She knows that all the nips, tucks, and good genes in the world can't make up for the positive mental mindset that comes with feeling fabulous. What a woman *is* on the inside will be what she exudes on the outside. For *her*, that's self-confidence and new energy. It's a certain glow and a pep in her step that gets her noticed wherever she goes. So if you are not feeling or acting like *her* right now, let's find out why.

Here's one way to look at it—by now, you're expert at many things in your personal and professional life. You are already fabulous. You are independent and in full control. You can solve problems for yourself, and you have greater emotional reliance. You are more aware of your strengths. You've accomplished things that have impacted countless people. Whether you know it or not, all of your life lessons and attributes make you a *Life Expert*. As a Life Expert, you can appreciate the wealth of experiences you've had.

Take Mama's Advice

Being a woman over sixty, I'm delighted when I hear the words, "You look great," or, "You look fabulous." This energizes me and makes my day. But if a day goes by and I'm "not feeling it," I remind myself of my own need for an attitude change—I think back to things Mama said that would make me feel better and helped shape who I am today.

I was born on the sunny island of Jamaica. I was raised by both parents, but it was Mama who always had a wise and wonderful way of looking at the world. Mama made me feel loved. Whenever I came home for visits, she would rush out to greet me, hugging me and telling me how proud she was of me. She had a big heart and always shared whatever she had with those who didn't have much.

Most of her sayings are difficult to translate from the Jamaican dialect, Patois, but the wisdom of her messages has helped me throughout my life. For instance, in Patois she would say: "When trouble ketch (catch) you, pickney (a child's) shut (shirt) fit you." Essentially what she meant was, when a problem arises, you've got to "make a child's shirt fit you"—in other words, recalibrate, dust yourself off, and keep going. Another one of her messages was, "Keep yu head up." Always carry yourself with dignity—something many mothers tell their children.

Although she wasn't college educated, Mama stressed the value of education—she always wanted me to work hard in school and excel academically. She emphasized that if you want something good out of life, you've got to put in the work. She was very proactive, believing, "Prevention is better than cure." In other words, be mindful and prevent problems from happening, rather than having to fix them later.

Over the years, I've found many of her sayings meaningful in my life, and today I pass on those same nuggets of wisdom to my daughter. In fact, just as many people "become their parents," I sometimes see my mother looking back at me when I look in the mirror today. She was tall and slim and dressed stylishly; she made many of her clothes herself as I did when I had the time. She had a pretty laugh and a great smile, which, combined with her statuesque appearance, really gave her a natural, earthy elegance.

Stay Healthy

When it comes to health, what's the difference between *her*—the woman who seems to have everything going for *her*—and you? She's taking care of herself. It's great to be fabulous, but you can't look or feel fabulous if unhealthy aging gets the best of you.

When Paula's mom, Maggie, turned eighty, Paula noticed that Maggie was becoming forgetful. Maggie needed help remembering simple things like taking her daily dose of blood pressure medicine and collecting the mail from her mailbox. Moving her to a nursing or assisted living home was out of the question, so Paula moved Maggie in to live with her. That's when Paula really saw firsthand the decline in Maggie's physical and mental health. Maggie could no longer take the stairs, and she needed help getting out of bed every morning; she was not the same vibrant, sassy woman who called the shots when she worked as a bank manager on Wall Street.

The change in Maggie was an awakening for Paula, who often joked with friends that she herself was about to turn the big "five-o" that year. But watching those glaring changes sparked questions about her own future. Paula wondered, *Will that be me in a few years? When is getting old going to catch up with me? Am I going to get Alzheimer's and not remember my name? Will I no longer be relevant? Who will take care of me?*

We all wish to live to a ripe, old age. Yet many middle-aged women fear aging. Let's face it, some of these fears aren't just about their health. They fear losing their youthful looks to sagging skin, bulging tummies, and thinning hair. They fear looking old and long to look young again.

The truth is, aging happens every day, and everyone ages. If you are among the women facing the fear of aging, this is the perfect time to change the conversation. The best way to quiet your fear of aging is to take matters into your own hands. Make this your turning point. Change course and dispel the negative stereotypes you have about aging.

The upcoming chapters will cover your mental, physical, and spiritual health.

For your mental health

Chapter 2, "**You Are Great—Share Your Best**," is about connecting to your community, taking pride in your age, sharing your talents, and mentoring the future. It shows how to perceive aging in a positive light and how to overcome fear and uncertainty. It can help you create a powerful vision of your future.

Chapter 3, "**Break Out of Your Comfort Zone**," tells you how to give yourself permission to roll out of your comfort zone and seek out things that nourish you.

Chapter 4, "**What's the Rush?**" shows how rushing can be an illusion, and focuses on meditation and peaceful routines.

For your physical health

Chapter 5, "**Beauty Beyond Fifty**," shows how to dial down your pace, turn back the clock, and look fabulous with good skin care**.**

Chapter 6, "**Nutrition—Eat for Life**," covers healthy eating for life, balancing calories, and maintaining a healthy weight.

Chapter 7, "**Exercise—A 'Good Thing**,'" shows how to incorporate physical activities to bolster a new and improved lifestyle, lower your risk for certain diseases, and ultimately extend your life.

Chapter 8, "**Health—Take Good Care of Yourself**," shows the importance of putting your health first, partnering with your health professional, and getting routine health screenings. The chapter covers managing stress and fueling your life with yoga and balance and strength exercises.

For your spiritual health

Chapter 9, "**Mindfulness—Give Thanks for the Rain, the Plants Need It**," shows how to truly give thanks for the rain, and how to find ways to find balance and care for your spirit.

Chapter 10, "**Affirmations—Think Positive**," delves into simple phrases or words that you can use to acknowledge and appreciate your personal attributes and situations to reinforce positive thoughts and feelings.

Chapter 11, "**Embrace the Tough Times**," shows that sometimes you need to pick yourself up and get on with life after a difficult situation. The Life Wheel exercises will give you a snapshot of how you are doing now.

When I caught up with Paula again a few months after her fiftieth birthday, I was curious about the health concerns that weighed heavily on her mind. Paula knew that although she couldn't prevent the changes that come with aging, there were things that she could control. "I've come to grips with being fifty. I can't guarantee that I won't become frail or get Alzheimer's like Mom," she said, "but I guarantee that I'll make the necessary lifestyle changes now for a better quality of life later."

Take Time to Embrace Your Best

So, you say you've led a busy and active life with your career and family. You've already proven your worth; nevertheless, you may feel that you still need to do more. This is the time to detox, recharge, travel at your leisure, take stay-cations, meet new people, sleep in, take leisurely walks, read long books, and be at ease. Essentially, you need to take time to enjoy life's simple pleasures. That's a lesson I learned one Saturday morning.

Naturally, on weekends, I like to get cozy and sleep late. But that Saturday morning, my Yorkshire Terrier, Bacardi, demanded I get up early, barking insistently as he stood at my bedside. So, I jumped out of bed—he can be very persistent when he wants to be taken out for a walk.

I slipped into comfortable clothes, laced up my sneakers, and dutifully took him out for his morning walk. When I returned a half-hour later, I thought that since I was already getting on with my morning, why not do some laundry. My oversized comforter needed to be laundered, but it wouldn't fit in my washing machine, so I took it to the laundromat a block away. Once it was in the washing machine, I had thirty minutes or so—enough time to get in a quick workout. So I hurried back to the private gym on the third floor of my apartment building. I did my usual exercise routine—a few minutes each on the elliptical, exercise bike, and treadmill, followed by a few rounds with ten-pound weights and finishing up with jumping jacks and yoga stretches.

After my workout, I dashed back to the laundromat just in time to catch the end of the wash cycle and put the comforter in the dryer. That gave me another thirty minutes to walk quickly to the supermarket two blocks away to buy my weekly stash of fresh fruits and vegetables. As I headed back to the laundromat from the supermarket to retrieve my very-dry comforter, I felt like I was on a TV reality show competing for first place to the finish line.

I reflected on my hurried morning and realized that although I accomplished a lot in an hour, I had not taken the time to enjoy the peaceful rhythm of a lovely weekend morning.

The truth is, you don't always have to be in motion. When you rush, you miss some awe-inspiring things—sights, sounds, and interactions with people. It's far better to be mindful and live in the moment, to savor your experiences, notice more, and appreciate things happening around you. So reclaim your weekends, sleep in, watch back-to-back episodes of your favorite shows. Take the time to embrace your best.

Remember Your Innate Confidence

Sometimes a woman over fifty needs help because of a setback in life. She may have lost faith in herself. She may have limiting beliefs—a fear of starting a new job or relationship, for example. She may fear being alone or having to depend on others. She may have financial uncertainties because she hasn't saved enough and her working years are coming to an end. She may fear the decline of her health and overall wellness, or she may just feel helpless.

If you find yourself in any of these circumstances, your ultimate goal must be to overcome your fear and create a positive and powerful vision of your future. Ask yourself, "What are my biggest fears? What's holding me back from overcoming these fears?" Then list what you need to do to overcome them. Create a realistic plan with measurable steps that let you see your progress as you work on your plan. Achieving the goals starts with getting rid of the things that block your progress. If you have a few missteps along the way, see them as teaching moments, and learn from them. Ask yourself, "What can I do differently the next time?" then get back on track.

Flip the Script

When you change the way you think and talk, you can begin to change the way you act. Use positive self-talk to turn "I can't" into "I can." Flipping the script means contradicting your negative internal dialogue with positive words and actions. For instance:

- Instead of saying, "I feel sad," say, **"I am alive, alert, awake, and enthusiastic."**

- Instead of saying, "I am afraid of speaking in public," say, **"I am an excellent, engaging speaker with something important to convey, and people listen intently to what I say."**

- Instead of saying, "I am depressed," say, **"Nothing can steal my joy. Today I experience things that make me happy."**

- Instead of saying, "I am stressed," say, **"I am calm, cool, and collected. I feel better with every breath I take."**

- Instead of saying, "I am afraid," say, **"I am bold, I am fearless, I am confident."**

chapter one takeaway

Being fabulous is so much more than superficial good looks. It means staying healthy and reclaiming time to rest and rejuvenate. It means a mindset makeover before a style makeover. It's time to leave fear and your old roles—mate, wife, employee, professional—behind. As a Life Expert, you can appreciate and use the wealth of experiences you've had. It's never too late to let yourself do more, to be strong, joyful, confident, in charge, and creative.

Exercises to Embrace Your Best Self

Advice for Your Over-Fifty Self
Every age has its own fears.
- What advice would you give yourself if you could go back and talk to your twenty-year-old self?

- Write down the advice.

- Is that the same advice you need now?

- What steps will you take to follow your advice?

The Mirror Exercise
The mirror exercise is a powerful tool that builds confidence. It teaches you to love what you see in the mirror. It can help you feel good about yourself and raise your self-esteem. All it takes is looking at your reflection and saying motivational statements to yourself.

You can try this exercise when you wake up in the morning, or just before you go to bed at night. Try it every day for thirty days and then for as often as you feel the need to do so.

1. You will need a mirror and a quiet, private space where you won't be disturbed.

2. Begin by looking into the mirror, and, for about ten minutes, speak kind phrases to yourself: "[*Your name*], I am so proud of you." "[*Your name*], you are the best." "[*Your name*], you are beautiful." Build on this, and make up your own inspirational phrases.

3. End the exercise by telling yourself, "[*Your name*], I love you."

Are you beginning to get the hang of it? Did it help you change how you feel about yourself?

chapter two

You Are Great—Share Your Best

Several years ago, Oprah Winfrey held an unforgettable walk in New York City. The theme of the walk was "Live Your Best Life."

Over thirty thousand walkers gathered on Mother's Day to raise money for several charities. I was a part of that walk. I watched as thousands of women of all ages eagerly made their way along the scenic bank of the Hudson River. The air was crisp that morning, and I could feel the excitement as my daughter and I scurried to try to find a good spot close to the music and festivities that kicked off the walk.

As an avid people watcher, I scanned the faces in the crowd. People seemed genuinely jubilant as they chatted and laughed with each other. Some took their exuberance a step further and danced to the music blaring overhead.

In the midst of it, I felt a sense of lightheartedness. I looked around and realized that many of the women in the crowd appeared to be like me—over fifty. Besides trying to get a close glimpse of Oprah, they all seemed to have one purpose—to "live their best life." As the walk got off to a brisk start, I felt pumped up and energized, and it dawned on me that the theme fit perfectly with the way I was feeling. It made me reflect on how free, unburdened, and wonderful life can be, especially when you share your experiences with others.

That moment was an epiphany for me. Like many people, I'd been living my life without really relishing in it. So, right then and there, I made the conscious decision to begin to live my version of my best life, by embracing my best. At first, it took some retraining to learn to take in and savor everyday moments, to live with intention and make the most out of my life. Today, I can actually *feel* the enjoyment I so deserve.

But what does it mean to "live your best life" or "embrace your best self"? Of course, the answer is different for everyone. For me, it's about focusing on what's good in my life and making the most of the present. I think of the things that have brought me the most joy and fulfillment: my health, my family, my daughter Antoinette, my dog Bacardi, my friends, a fun vacation, great food, and the kindness of others. Looking at this list, it's clear that what brings out the best in me are the moments and experiences shared with others. This is true for most of us—we embrace our best if we share our best.

Take Alex, who at fifty-five works as an administrative assistant in a Brooklyn law office. For Alex, embracing her best means appreciating the opportunities and experiences she has had with other people. She doesn't take the people in her life for granted. Often she reaches out to friends to invite them to join her at social events. She exudes warmth, and she takes the time to compliment others. She chooses to be happy by looking on the bright side and finding the silver lining wherever she can. Each day, she reflects on the good around her. Most importantly, she shares her best by mentoring teenage girls in her Big Sister group. She looks forward to working with the girls twice a month, and helping them realize their full potential. No doubt her work has a lasting impact.

Sharing your best is about connecting. It's connecting to a community, large or small, and sharing your talents to mentor the future. You can share your best in three ways—*engaging with others, building a network,* and *starting anew every day.*

Engage with Others

Discovering and sharing your best comes from engaging with others. There is great power in a community of women coming together, whether socially or for business. I saw this first-hand growing up in Jamaica. The close-knit community I lived in, Savanna-La Mar (translation: "plains by the sea"), had British, African, and Spanish roots. At that time, we were a British colony, so our education was similar to that in the schools of England. We enjoyed school, learning about colonization, reciting Shakespeare, participating in competitive sports—cricket, football, and Olympic-style track-and-field activities—and watching free outdoor movies on the school grounds on Friday nights. On weekends, we frequented the white-sand beaches nearby, but not before we got stern warnings from our parents to, "Be careful not to drown." We had an abundance of mango, orange, and plum trees, so it was easy to reach up on tiptoe and pick fruits when they were in season. I still remember what a treat it was to eat freshly cut, juicy sugarcane that came straight from our backyard.

Most of all, I remember how the women in our community looked out for each other through thick and thin. They cared about their neighbors and extended a helping hand to those in need. They had strong social connections, so there was always someone to bounce ideas off and give advice. Whenever someone was ill, a neighbor would come calling with dinner, sparing the family the burden of having to cook. I saw this firsthand when my dad was ill. Our neighbor Miss Wilson and her daughter Mazie showed up regularly with steamed red snapper dinners that were out-of-this-world.

The older women in the community were the caretakers who babysat for free—old-fashioned daycare—and gave advice on just about everything, including folk medicine and cures for all kinds of maladies. I heard them talk often about *cerasee*, a bitter, leafy, vine that grew wild on fences and shrubs. The women would say, "A *cerasee* bath will clear up your skin," or, "What you need is some good strong *cerasee* tea to cleanse your blood." Likewise, they swore by the *leaf of life*, a wild succulent plant used as a cure for the common cold, fever, and respiratory illness. They would advise, "Beat (pound) the leaves, extract the juice, add a little sugar or salt, and drink it."

It's refreshing to engage with other women and create an inner circle, just as these women did. It can be meeting girlfriends for brunch, yoga, bowling, or a ceramics class. When you spend time with others—individuals or in communities—you will begin to build connections, learn new things, and have new experiences. The key is, when you meet someone new, make it a point to exchange contact information—for professional connections, exchange business cards. If you are tech savvy, scan quick response (QR) codes using your smartphone and instantly share information. Then follow up using email, phone, or social media within a couple of days. Initiate regular check-ins, or meet for coffee, tea, drinks, lunch, brunch—but stick to the plan and just do it.

Expand Your Network

Often, well-meaning people will say, "Let's meet for coffee sometime!" but it never happens. The next time they meet, they'll say, "We still have to go for coffee!" They're simply being polite, or just haven't gotten around to it. Getting together for coffee is a great way to begin building a network of connections—powerful, but far less complicated than you think.

People play different roles in each other's lives—that's especially true for women. Some women have a small and tight circle of friends. Others have different circles of friends for shopping, going to the theater, book club, jogging in the park, visiting each other for potlucks, or just sitting and chatting about this and that. The circles may even include men. Usually, these circles are made up of a select group of friends who they'll tell everything—the good, the bad, and the ugly.

So find other people to be with—whether it makes sense to start or join a book club, a walking group, a community garden, meet-ups, or an advocacy group working for some kind of social change. Often, new friendships will develop out of these networking opportunities—book clubs, for instance, are notorious for being places where the book discussion takes a back seat to the social interaction. The group will spend an hour getting caught up before someone finally says, "Okay. Now we've *really* got to talk about the book."

Expanding your network will help you make new acquaintances and get the scoop on hot happenings around town, giving you access to information you are not likely to get elsewhere. For instance, when someone in my book club mentioned a New York Philharmonic *Concerts in the Parks* performance in Central Park, I wasn't about to miss out, so like everyone else I showed up with my snacks and blanket. Let's be honest—something as amazing as an afternoon in the park is much more exciting to talk about with friends than gallstones or an aching back.

Longtime friends and far-away relatives can also be part of your network. It's common for relationships that were once very strong to become distant over time. How about those cousins or childhood friends you see only at family reunions, holidays, weddings, and funerals? If you've grown apart and you still care for them, rekindle those friendships beyond special occasions.

Now that everyone has access to social media, it's easy to start and continue long-distance friendships or look up friends from the past. Many people have successfully reconnected with folks they've lost touch with over the years. In fact, I've seen some of those reconnections actually end up with marriage proposals.

Start Anew Every Day

Living and sharing your best is as simple as remembering your new direction from the moment you get out of bed. Remind yourself to feel good about yourself, be euphoric about life, and spread the feeling around.

Let me share with you a story about starting anew. Remember in chapter 1, when I mentioned my experience with my new empty nest? It happened when my daughter, Antoinette, left for college. Although I was proud and happy for her, I did not realize the void I would feel while she was away at school.

When she finished college, I thought she would move back home indefinitely. She was always a go-getter, very self-confident, and sociable, but it never dawned on me that she might be ready to build her own life as an independent adult away from the home we lived in for many years.

After college, she returned home to New York, and before long she got a job. In the evenings, I looked forward to picking her up at the bus stop. On Sundays, I cooked her favorite foods, and we would have family dinners and watch TV together. I was always excited about the time we spent together, and I enjoyed catching up and hearing the latest news about her friends and work.

It wasn't long before she was soft-selling me on the idea of getting her own apartment in Manhattan. Each day, I watched with a sinking feeling as she surfed the internet and showed me pictures of apartments she liked. I was happy that she was launching out on her own, but I dreaded the time when she would be living elsewhere and I wouldn't see her every day. As you can probably tell, my daughter is my best friend, and we really enjoy each other's company.

At last, one day she asked me to accompany her to look at apartments. Within a day, we found an apartment in a desirable area on the Upper West Side of Manhattan. It was ingenious of her to include me in her apartment hunting—I too got caught up in the excitement of helping her search and pick out new furniture. It made the letdown of her leaving a lot easier.

That first week after she left was lonely. I began to wonder, "Will we get to see each other on a regular basis?" Then I came up with what turned out to be a brilliant idea. I suggested we set aside one night a week to do something special together—a "date night" of sorts. We decided that on Friday evenings we would get together and do something we both enjoyed. Even though we talked on the phone throughout the week, Fridays became quite exciting because we knew we'd see each other. During the day, we made plans, deciding what we were going to do and where we were going to meet. My own excitement spilled over into my office so much that on Fridays my coworkers would ask, "What are you and Antoinette doing this evening?"

Most of the time, we had dinner at a restaurant and would spend hours just chatting and laughing, and we took turns picking up the tab at the end of the night. We'd cap the evening off by walking to Times Square, where we would sit under the bold lights and just people watch.

Although I gave her an "out" by telling her that we could skip our date night whenever she had something really important to do, we rarely missed date night for the first few years. Nowadays, even if we don't have a regular date night, we still manage to get together every week.

Plan date nights with your kids if you live within close proximity. The date nights with my daughter helped me bridge the gap of living alone in a big house after she moved out. If you are far away, set time aside to call, and use social media like Facebook or Instagram, or Skype or FaceTime, to stay in touch. We have one rule for date night though—it must be fun. No groaning about work, and no complaining about aches and pains.

Interestingly, my daughter's move inspired me to eventually sell my house in the suburbs and move to the city—much closer to her—I'll discuss this more in chapter 3.

Spend Time with People Older and Younger Than You

There is something very soothing and calming about talking to someone older and wiser than yourself. Older people are great storytellers. Listening to stories told by older people has a way of transporting you to another place in time. Often the stories are about their life experiences, told in rich, vivid terms—stories you can relate to and learn from.

Likewise, as you get older, you can give back by sharing your own stories and life experiences with younger people. While your body may be changing, one thing that won't change are the life experiences you've had. You are equipped to give solace, sagely advice, and your own perspective on life. It is gratifying and empowering to have someone look to you for your knowledge and wisdom.

Frankly, one of the delightful things that many middle-aged women experience is the vitality and youthfulness that comes from being around younger people. The fact is, we are living much longer, so there is plenty of opportunity for women to get involved in the lives of younger generations.

If you have grandchildren, it can be energizing to be actively involved in their lives. My friend, Bev, dotes on her five-year-old granddaughter, Kylie. Bev proudly tells her friends about the smart things Kylie always says and the amazing questions she asks as they putter around the house together. If you don't have grandchildren, you can have the same experience with the children of your friends and family.

Some people say "age is just a number," and I agree. Age is something to celebrate. Amy is a great example of someone who embraces her age and shares that excitement with friends and family. When she turned sixty, she threw herself a big birthday bash at a hotel in town. She arrived at the party looking radiant in a crimson, figure-hugging gown. As I signed her guest book, I couldn't help but be impressed with the huge turnout. I was not at all surprised at the accolades and acknowledgments she received that night.

Five years later at age sixty-five, Amy announced she was retiring from her job as the director of business development at a media company. This time, she gave herself a retirement dinner. Surrounded by family and friends, she looked happy, flaunting the fact that she was finally "hanging up her nine-to-five hat." These days she is busy as a bee, volunteering on her local community board. There's good news for Amy, because research shows that volunteering reduces mortality risk by 25 percent.[2] Amy is enjoying her nieces and nephews and traveling to places she'd never been. She stays connected with family and friends through text messaging, e-cards, emails, and weekend brunches. Her most recent email came with pictures proudly announcing that her grandniece, Mercedes, had just turned five.

Amy takes pride in her age; she proves that even as she ages, she is no slouch. Instead of being fearful and apprehensive, she is courageous, celebrates all that she is, appreciates all that she has, and is doing all that she can do. Most of all, she is involved in the lives of younger people. The physical changes in her body have not stopped her. She has not made the stereotypes about aging deter her. Instead, she channels this into activities that speak deeply to her love for life.

---

2   M.A. Okun, E.W. Young, and S. Brown, "Volunteering by older adults and risk of mortality: A meta-analysis." *Psychol. Aging*, Jun 2013; 28(2):564-577. doi: 10.1037/a0031519. Epub 2013 Feb 18, https://www.ncbi.nlm.nih.gov/m/pubme d/23421326/?i=4&from=/23545605/related.

Share Your Talents

Many women have hidden talents, talents that they've not shared with others. What talents do you have to share?

Do you play a musical instrument—the piano, perhaps? Do you sing, write? Are you good at interior design? Are you a foodie, a whiz in the kitchen? Are you naturally nurturing? Are you technologically or business savvy? Your talents can be of real value if you share them with someone else.

Take stock of what life has taught you, and the wisdom you've gained from your personal experiences. What can you offer that can influence and enrich someone else's life?

I grew up with an affinity for do-it-yourself tricks like picking out paint colors at the hardware store, painting a room in my house, mounting wall hangings, and designing and sewing my own clothes. Today, if a dress is too long, I know how to shorten it. If it's loose fitting, I know how to make it fit. In fact, my daughter was fascinated the first time I showed her a few simple hand-sewing techniques to fix the fraying hem on a skirt.

Nothing beats the touch and feel of hands-on learning, like making something from scratch, like baking a cake or making a special dish. A skill that you may feel is ordinary or commonplace could be of great value to someone young and less experienced.

Even with hands-on learning, there are those "phone-a-friend" instances that inevitably happen. How often do we hear of a newlywed picking up the phone to call a parent to walk them through a recipe as they cook the

> **A skill that you may feel is ordinary or commonplace could be of great value to someone young and less experienced.**

first meal for their spouse, or host their first party? Or how about the calls to save a recipe when they forgot an important ingredient? That's just what happened when Karen, one of Antoinette's friends, invited her over for dinner.

Antoinette arrived at Karen's house to find her in a panic. It seems that just before she put the pie in the oven, Karen realized she had forgotten to put in eggs. In a last-minute ditch to save dessert, Karen made a "lifeline" call to her father, who told her to simply scoop all the filling from the pie shell into a mixing bowl, whip in the eggs, pour it back into the shell, and pop it into the oven. Thankfully, the pie was saved and dinner was a success.

Sharing your talents with others can have a ripple effect that is far-reaching. As word gets out, a much larger circle of people may learn something new because of you. Think of it this way: You have many life lessons under your belt. When you share these life lessons with others, you become a *Life Teacher*.

So, consider the talents you have that can benefit others. What can you share that might help them, and that they can use to ultimately help even more people?

Mentor the Future

When you mentor someone, you are paying it forward—giving back to society. You are a role model, helping another person fill gaps in their life experience. Over the years, people have turned to me for advice, inspiring me to now mentor others.

One of the early moments when I realized that I had an aptitude for mentoring happened when one of my associates kept nudging her daughter to talk with me. Her daughter was considering a career change, and although I didn't see myself as a career counselor, when she emailed me to arrange a meeting, I agreed. Within weeks, I had agreed to mentor a colleague who was contemplating law school versus accepting a lucrative position as operations manager in her company. Since then, I have been a mentor to several others on personal and career matters.

Mentoring and coaching are ways you can use your gifts to give back to others. A mentor or coach can help others discover, clarify, and realign their personal or professional goals. That's why I signed on as a mentor with American Corporate Partners (ACP), a nonprofit organization that helps veterans prepare for their next step in a career after the military service. I mentor these individuals before they transition into the civilian workforce. Each mentorship relationship typically lasts a year.

I am proud to say that one of my former protégés is now an officer in the Marines. When he called me with this good news, he was leaving to begin work in Japan. My most recent protégé was deployed to Africa, so we scheduled monthly phone calls to work on his professional strengths.

In contrast to mentoring, as a coach I help the coachee find answers and generate their own strategies. For example, when I'm talking with someone who is trying to resolve an issue, and they suddenly have an *aha!* moment—a light bulb moment when something becomes clear—I'll get them to pause and dig even deeper. A life coach knows when and how to ask probing questions, like, "Tell me more about that," "How did that make you feel?" or, "What do you want to get out of this session today?" By delving deeper, coachees often find themselves on a path to self-discovery and finding solutions on their own.

As a coach, I serve as a mirror of sorts to help others reflect on what they already know. I can give them the tools they need by simply asking the right questions, empowering them to find their true potential as they try to create and fulfill their goals and desires.

It is gratifying to be able to use your experience to help others, and to pay it forward. When other people ask you for help, it will make you feel good about your own level of maturity and remind you of what you have to offer.

Be There for Others by Listening

Sharing your best can be just being present and actively listening, especially if you know that someone is going through a rough patch. Giving them your time and attention can be the best gift you can offer.

For instance, starting a new romantic relationship later in life may be unnerving and difficult for some women. This is true particularly if one of the partners has adult children who object. If a friend comes to you feeling torn between loyalty to her children and her desire to be with a new love, then listening without hastening to "weigh in" is first and foremost.

The same situation often happens in reverse—a friend may feel that her needs are being ignored by her partner for the sake of his adult children. This sounds like Maxine's story. Her relationship with the man she deeply cared for was under a lot of strain. At sixty years old, she felt her interests had taken a backseat, because he made it clear that his son and teenage grandson came first. She was unsure about the future of their relationship. I have seen similar situations with other couples rebound, so I didn't want her to lose hope and throw in the towel. Instead of judging or offering advice, I left the door open for her to decide for herself—and gave it time. "Do you want it to work?" I asked. "Have you met to talk things through?"

As you might have guessed, Maxine said, "I want it to work with all my heart."

Well, they did meet. They hashed things out, and both sides got a better understanding of each other's boundaries and priorities. After a few get-togethers and family outings, Maxine got to know his son and grandson better. She no longer felt left out. She told me that with everyone's blessings, they were happy and taking things to the next level and talking about getting married that spring.

Artful listening involves knowing when to listen and when to share. It's tempting to hijack the conversation and jump in to tell someone your own story, simply to confirm that you understand. On occasion, listening means being vulnerable and sharing a story from your own life experience; this helps others know that you understand what they are going through. But first listen to what the person is saying, and nod or give a verbal hint to let them know that you heard and understand what they said. Listen mostly for cues to what they really want from you. Do they even want advice from you, or do they just want to be heard?

So create a safe place where someone can open up and express their thoughts and feelings and ideas—but mostly just listen.

chapter two takeaway

Shared joy is palpable, and it's contagious, just like the Oprah walk. Share your best by building partnerships, staying in touch, and surrounding yourself with people who make you feel positive and uplifted. Love and care for yourself so that you can be there to love and care for someone else. Stay physically and socially active by being connected to a circle or community. A good inner circle is energizing. Whether you're mentoring or coaching someone, you're really sharing your talents and building relationships.

An Exercise for Embracing Your Best Self

Sharing Your Best Gift
List four gifts or talents that you have to share with others.

1. _____

2. _____

3. _____

4. _____

chapter three

Break Out of Your Comfort Zone

After having lived away from city life for over twenty years, I decided to go back. I had originally moved to the suburbs with my young daughter after the passing of my husband. For years, I missed the excitement and social opportunities that living in the city offered, mostly because I had grown comfortable with suburban life. Three years after my daughter left home and moved to the city, I took the plunge and left isolation behind. I broke out of my comfort zone and followed her and my heart back to the city.

Despite being somewhat apprehensive about being out and about by myself in the big city, I left the comfort of the suburbs behind. It helped that I fell in love with the apartment my realtor showed me. It was everything I wanted: a location on a quiet street, lots of windows with natural light, great views, a nice rooftop garden space for relaxing and entertainment, a private gym, and only a ten-minute train ride to work.

I knew very little about the surrounding neighborhoods, so one Saturday morning I donned my walking shoes, gathered up enough courage, and ventured out to explore. I walked along the street where I live and headed west, toward the sounds of people and traffic. I came to a busy intersection, which turned out to be the iconic Malcolm X Boulevard. I decided to turn left and kept walking. To my delight, I saw treetops in the distance—it was a park. As I drew closer, I realized that I had inadvertently come upon the north side of Central Park. I had been living in the city for a couple of months now, but didn't know that my apartment was within walking distance of Central Park North.

When I realized what I had stumbled upon, I began to take it all in. There was a flurry of activity around me: people walking, jogging, and riding bikes. Some were with family and friends, others were walking their dogs, and some were just sitting on the grass or on park benches peacefully enjoying the morning.

"Wow," I thought, "*this* is the place to be!" This charming section of the park that sits between Fifth Avenue and Central Park West screamed, "Look at me in all of my natural element." There was a lake near the entrance to the park, and as I gazed into the water, I saw tiny turtles floating, their heads slowly breaking the surface and then quickly disappearing underwater. Here and there I saw families of ducks—with mama ducks dutifully watching their adorable offsprings as they proudly paraded along the bank.

As I ventured further into the park, I saw water gushing from a nearby waterfall. I absorbed the gentle, relaxing sounds. I inched toward a group of people curiously gazing at something and taking pictures. *It must be something special*, I thought—and I was right. It was the park's lily pond in the English garden. This hidden gem was full of elegant floating pink and purple blooms. For me, it was an enchanting moment.

I wandered through the manicured gardens and began looking at the plants. I marveled at the ornamental zebra grasses and colorful flowers, and I touched the tiny leaves of some plants I'd never seen before. I began to experience the park in all its splendor, discovering beauty at every turn.

Since that day, I was hooked. On weekends, when I have no other plans, I head for the park to reboot my spirit. Sometimes I join the throngs of runners for a quick run, visit my favorite spots, or just sit on a bench and absorb the openness and fresh air.

Discovering the park opened my eyes. I've found that there are all sorts of free activities happening all the time. My personal favorites include the outdoor Concerts in the Parks series on the Great Lawn, and the Shakespeare in the Park performances. I now show up with my blanket and food, enjoying the performances with other people.

There's a certain amount of excitement and payback that comes from going to events like these. Wherever you live, especially if you are in a big, bustling city like New York City, finding new activities to enjoy can have a grounding effect. It can make you feel connected to the rest of the world—something bigger than yourself.

When I'm sitting on the grass in Central Park, surrounded by city life and listening to beautiful music, I can't help but look back and think: how did I arrive here? The only answer I have is that I left my comfort zone behind for unknown but new and amazing experiences.

You Don't Have to Be Alone

Women in middle age may sometimes find themselves feeling lonely and isolated, feelings so firmly entrenched that it's difficult for them to make a change. At this time in your life, you don't have to sit at home and be lonely.

Making changes later in life is not always easy. The decision to make a big change—like moving—won't happen overnight. For me, it took time to actually decide: I had a nice house with trees, a beautiful lawn, and a garden. It was in a quiet neighborhood where I could grow things and listen to birds chirping or look out my kitchen window and see rabbits hopping about and deer roaming across the lawn. Great shopping and a church were nearby, and I could get to work by car or express bus within an hour.

But I realized that my social life was dwindling. Networks of friends in the suburbs are often spread out, and the friendships built when raising our families often dissipate after the kids are gone. You no longer live vicariously through their activities. I'd often leave work in a rush to get the express bus or drive home to an empty house, where I'd spend the evening watching television. I'd wake up refreshed the next morning, and start my routine all over again, with very little "quality" time during the week.

Yet, there comes a time in midlife where downsizing and a change of scenery begin to sound enticing. This, however, is not always easy. It's not easy to get rid of things you're attached to. Many of the things you own have sentimental value. It's a big—and often very difficult—decision to give up your "white picket fence."

Make New Experiences

Begin to break out of your comfort zone by first weighing the pros and cons of your life now, and the pros and cons of the changes you want to make. What are your best options? What will make you happy, and at what cost?

For instance, if you make the decision to downsize and move to a new place, can you find things in your new surroundings that interest you? For me, the park was a great substitute for my pleasant backyard. I was drawn to the beautiful flowers, and by touching their petals and leaves. I felt a connection to the garden I used to have. When I saw the lake, I was excited, and connected it to the lakes I used to visit upstate.

So, look on the bright side. Although it may be a bit uncomfortable at first, step outside of your comfort zone. You may discover things that bring you pleasure and help you love your new surroundings even more.

Look for new things to do. Learn to swim, take a dance class, get theater tickets, go to the movies, or connect with an organization. When I moved back to the city, one of the first things I did was to join the Lincoln Center. Now I get exclusive benefits like seeing the newest performances at discounted prices and getting show tickets in advance well before the general public.

If you are unsure about how to take that first step outside your routine, invite a friend or family member to join you. If you're concerned about going out at night, look for daytime activities. In New York, for instance, there are affordable matinees that attract many middle-aged people. Every city has affordable or free activities if you just look for them. Your local visitor's center can be a great help in finding free, fun events to help you break out of your comfort zone.

Take a Girls' Weekend Trip

Breaking out of your comfort zone means taking a leap and doing something entirely new, and that's precisely what happened when one of my colleagues suggested that we get together with another colleague for a girls' weekend trip. We jumped at the opportunity because she owned a home in Massachusetts near a yoga center that she often raved about. We would stay at her home, tour the yoga center, and visit the small town nearby. We decided on the weekend, and that Friday after work we piled our snacks and weekend bags into her car and headed for Massachusetts, chatting nonstop the entire way.

The next morning, we woke early to a glorious sunrise on the horizon, so we went for a brisk walk around the town, where we had brunch at a café and visited a farmer's market. Afterwards, we headed over to the yoga center for a tour, a mostly vegan dinner, and an evening concert. We drove back home on Sunday afternoon after a great weekend, making plans for our next trip.

We had never gone on a girls' weekend trip together before, but all it took was a bright idea from one person and setting the date to make it happen.

These days, girls' weekend getaways are increasingly popular. Breaking outside your comfort zone and taking a trip with friends is a great way to connect with others, to build new friendships, and strengthen existing ones. You can pamper yourselves by taking advantage of retreat packages with activities ranging from relaxing spa days to gliding amongst the trees on a thrilling zip line.

Get Out of Your Way

You'll always have reasons why you stay in your comfort zone. It is easy to tell yourself, "I don't have the time," "I don't have the money," or, "I feel guilty or selfish when I do something nice for myself." But your excuses are only putting obstacles in your way.

For a long time, fifty-five-year-old Lisa wanted to go back to school to pursue a degree in early childhood education. Her irregular work schedule as a retail associate made it difficult to carve out time for school. But she also nursed nagging memories of the time her high school teacher told her that she was "not the brightest crayon in the box." Her fear of failure made her put off going back to school. Who was going to pay the tuition? Would her boss change her work schedule so that she could take evening classes? Was she too old to go back to school or even start a new career?

After much prodding from her friend, Leann, Lisa finally spoke to a college career counselor, who helped her map out the steps to qualify for admission. A year later, Lisa was ready. She got into the program, qualified for financial aid, and even managed to negotiate a new work schedule with her boss. She had finally gotten out of her own way. For years, she had wrestled with inner chaos and self-doubt. She felt that she was not good enough to get into college, and that the college application process was too tedious. Yet, she got out of her own way, took the leap, and sought advice. All the while, she pictured rewards of a better work-life balance, a better paying job, and the fulfillment of a longtime dream.

When you are in your fifties, sixties, and beyond, it's likely that you have more freedom now to do things you didn't have the chance to do before. Whether you are exploring a new experience, a career change, or contemplating a life-changing decision, think about the long-term benefits. All you need to do is get out of your own way.

Getting out of your way means not putting up self-sabotaging, self-defeating roadblocks that prevent you from doing things you wish you could do. On the surface, my visits to the park and the girls' weekend trip seemed ordinary, but they were rewarding. I found beauty and charm in the park, the small town, the yoga center, and the farmer's market. All of which restored and grounded me once I got of my own way.

Getting out of your way means not putting up self-sabotaging, self-defeating road-blocks that prevent you from doing things you wish you could do.

Age Happy, Live Happy

Admittedly, living happy is something many people have difficulty sustaining from one day to the next. Allowing yourself to experience happiness is a choice you can consciously make. One study of over three hundred thousand adults found that the ages sixty-five to seventy-nine are the happiest ages.[3]

Interestingly enough, a number of studies on happiness have uncovered many benefits of mental and physical health. Harvard University professor Tal Ben-Shahar created a course on happiness that has become one of the university's most popular courses.[4] In Positive Psychology 1504, Ben-Shahar teaches that happiness is not an accident. He says we should live in the moment and make the most of our lives.

---

3   Matthew Steel, "Measuring National Well-being: At what age is Personal Well-being the highest?" Office for National Statistics, February 2016, https://www.ons.gov.uk/peoplepopulationandcommunity/wellbeing/articles/measuringnationalwellbeing/atwhatageispersonalwellbeingthehighest.

4   Fabrega, Marelisa, "Harvard's most popular course: Tal Ben-Shahar on how to be happier," Daring to Live Fully, accessed June 1, 2017, https://daringtolivefully.com/happier-tal-ben-shahar.

Even the smiley face that was so popular in the 1970s has evolved into social media's lively emoticons and emojis, many conveying varying degrees of happiness. Numerous seminars, books, and songs have been created around the fascinating pursuit of happiness. Among the songs, my favorite is "Happy" by Pharrell, and you might remember the song "Don't Worry, Be Happy" by Bobby McFerrin. With happiness comes laughter. Laughter is truly *good medicine*, and programs have been developed to get the blood pumping through laughter. One of the more interesting of these is laughter yoga, where the participants stare at each other and keep laughing.

Boost Your Mood

One way to boost your mood is to increase your levels of *serotonin* and *endorphins*, which are "feel good" neurotransmitters, or chemical messengers, in your body. Serotonin is believed to play a role in several physical and psychological functions that make you feel good. Low levels of serotonin are responsible for mood imbalance, anxiety, loneliness, and depression. High levels have the opposite effect, making you feel good. You can increase your serotonin levels with more sunlight, exercise, and with foods like dark chocolate, oats, dried dates, milk, yogurt, cottage cheese, eggs, fish, chick peas, almonds, and sunflower seeds. Endorphins also give you sensations of well-being, making you feel good and laugh more.

In chapter 7, I will discuss how a daily exercise routine will not only enhance your fitness and energy levels, but also help to increase your serotonin and endorphin levels and improve your mood. Another way to boost your mood is sunlight. A little sunlight is not only nature's way of helping to increase the levels of vitamin D in your body, but it can also boost your mood. Researchers at Cornell University studying the effects of windows and daylight found that hospital nurses who were exposed to natural light in their work settings communicated more and laughed more than those who worked in areas that were not lit by natural light.[5] So, let the sunshine in and spend more daylight time in natural light or outdoors to boost your mood.

---

5   Rana Sagha Zadeh, et al., "The impact of windows and daylight on acute-care nurses' physiological, psychological, and behavioral health, *Health Environments Research & Design Journal* 7, no. 4 (Summer 2014): 35-61.

chapter three takeaway

Get emotionally ready to enjoy life. Break outside your comfort zone—you could find a far more fabulous and rewarding world awaiting you. Once you embrace the fact that you're getting older, you can begin to find ways to truly live happy. What's important is living your life to the fullest. You become what you live. When you choose to live happy, you age happy.

An Exercise to Embrace Your Best Self

Breaking Out of Your Comfort Zone

1. What have you been putting on hold?

   _____

2. What will you do to change this?

   _____

3. When will you do it?

   _____

4. What one limiting belief prevents you from getting out of your comfort zone?

   _____

5. What do you need to do to get rid of your limiting belief?

   _____

chapter four

What's the Rush?

New Yorkers get a bad rap for always being in a hurry. We're always rushing from place to place as if everything must be done *yesterday*. Going through life with too much on our plate and too little time is especially true for some women—whether in a big city or a small town.

You've probably said it many times: "If only the day had more than twenty-four hours, I'd be able to get everything done!" There's always something for us to schedule or check off on our to-do list. Take fifty-six-year-old Roni, a business manager for a large retail chain. This is what her typical morning looks like:

7:00 a.m. – Alarm clock rings. Roni springs out of bed. Both feet hit the floor. She rushes around her apartment getting dressed, doing her hair, putting on makeup, getting ready for work.

8:00 a.m. – Sprints out the door. She's on a mission to make the next train, so she picks up speed, fearing she might miss it.

8:15 a.m. – Dashes down the steps of the subway as the speaker overhead announces a train is approaching the station. She steps aboard just before the doors close.

8:45 a.m. – Hustles off the train. Makes a quick stop at Starbucks to pick up a latte. Standing in line, she realizes she left her phone on her nightstand. She mentally goes over her to-do list for the day. First, a 9:00 a.m. meeting, where she's on the agenda to give a monthly financial report to the management team.

9:00 a.m. – Arrives at the office. An account executive needs her help. She quickly answers his question, grabs the financial report from her desk and heads to the meeting.

9:05 a.m. – Enters the meeting room. She's dismayed to find no one there. Then she realizes she is in the wrong room.

9:15 a.m. – Finally finds the meeting room and joins the meeting— fifteen minutes late. Shuffling through her papers, she realizes that she mistakenly grabbed last month's report. Anxiety begins to set in, as she offers her apologies for not having the correct report.

10:00 a.m. – Now back in her office, Roni slumps in her chair in despair. Although the day has just started, she is already worn. She wonders, how did this happen?

The truth is, many working women start their day like Roni—in a hurry. From their first step out of bed, every minute is programmed, every move on autopilot. The dog (if there is one) has to be walked. Lunchtime is a hurried break, or is taken at their desk. Evenings are packed with all sorts of activities. The clock ticks away as they attend to one time-sensitive pursuit after another: meetings, projects, family commitments, important dates. The pace is rush, rush, rush. And that rush becomes a pattern.

By the time you've reached middle age, your responsibilities should be more pared down, even if you are still in the workforce. If they're not, then it's time to embrace simplicity. Take a closer look to see if the things you're doing are really necessary. Pull back and reassess what's important. It's time to cut the stress, avoid things that are unnecessary, and replace them with things that are meaningful. Ask yourself, "What can I eliminate from my day and still do what needs to be done?" "What am I doing that is no longer necessary?" "What should I start or continue doing to bring me more peace?"

By deciding what's important, you can begin to find ways to dial down your pace. Instead of chaos, a sense of calm sets the tone for your entire day.

Begin with a Peaceful Morning Routine

My morning starts calmly by reading something positive and inspirational. Some of my favorite authors are Louise Hay, Cheryl Richardson, Ruth Fishel, Catherine Ponder, Joel Osteen, Florence Scovel Shinn, Christiane Northrup, and Sarah Ban Breathnach. After reading, I meditate for a few minutes until my mind starts to wander. Next I head to the gym for my twenty- to thirty-minute workout. Back from the gym, I brush my dog Bacardi's hair—he doesn't like it, but I tell him, "We've got to get ready. We've got to get you nice and handsome." Looking well groomed, he's ready for a quick walk—he loves going out. All this is part of my morning ritual, just like showering and getting dressed. It makes me ready to face the day with a healthy attitude.

Having a good morning ritual can center and give you a feeling of serenity all day long. It prepares you to better handle stress and any unexpected crises that comes your way. Done right, those few minutes in the morning can make your whole day more peaceful—and more productive.

So start each day by taking a moment to center yourself to decide on the things you need to do. Develop your own peaceful routine, one that makes you feel like you just did something good for yourself. What better way to start the day?

Rely On Your Own Rhythm

One way to start your day with calm instead of chaos is to train yourself to wake naturally. After a while, you will be conditioned to wake up around the same time each morning, without being jarred awake by a blaring alarm clock. If an alarm is a must, then set it fifteen to twenty minutes ahead of the time you want to wake. Use those few extra minutes in bed to leisurely reflect on the day ahead.

Get Your "Happy Hormones" Going

After your fifteen minutes of reflection, get up and get your body moving. Start with a few stretches and exercises to wake up your body and your mind. Exercise boosts your energy and triggers *endorphins*—the "feel-good" neurotransmitters we discussed in the previous chapter. One study found that low-intensity exercise reduced fatigue by 65 percent and raised energy levels by 20 percent.[6]

---

6   Sam Fahmy, "Low-intensity exercise reduces fatigue symptoms by 65 percent, study finds," UGA Today, February 28, 2008, accessed April 18, 2017, http://news.uga.edu/releases/article/low-intensity-exercise-reduces-fatigue-symptoms-by-65-percent-study-finds/.

Even doing light or low-intensity exercise can help—something as easy as walking, stretching, or simple yoga can be effective. There's more to come on exercise and yoga in chapters 8 and 9.

Read or Write Something Positive

Start your day with good thoughts. As you sip your morning cup of coffee or tea, read something inspirational: a quote, an affirmation, the verse of the day, a prayer, or something from a motivational book. Writing in a gratitude journal or doing the mirror exercise from chapter 1 can also set a positive tone for your day.

Plan Better

Planning ahead lessens the chances of things spiraling out of control. At night, review your schedule for the next day. What will you eat? What's tomorrow's weather forecast? What will you wear? Will you need an umbrella or rain gear? No need for surprises when you step outdoors.

You have many competing demands in a day, so prioritize and ask yourself, "Which of these things are *must-dos* today? Which adds value? What happens if I don't do something today?" You might find yourself getting caught up in deciding what's really important.

I found this out recently when I was preparing to go to a friend's wedding. The decisions about what to wear became a big deal at the last minute. I had planned to wear a short dress, but when my daughter Antoinette suggested that I wear an evening gown, everything changed. First, I had to choose which gown to wear, and which shoes—my fancy, three-inch blinged-out pair of heels, or a more comfortable pair perfect for dancing at the reception? Which purse was large enough to hold my lipstick, powder, and reading glasses?

How should I style my hair? What color nail polish? and so on. I spent more than an hour trading text messages and photos of dresses and shoes with Antoinette and my friend, Liz, trying to agree on what to wear. But I still hadn't made a decision.

Then there was the real dilemma: what jewelry to wear. At that point, I thought I still had time to run out and pick up new earrings. Frankly, I have plenty of earrings and didn't need a new pair for the occasion. But for a moment I was convinced I needed the perfect set to complement the rose-gold dress I'd picked out. I thought, while I'm at it, I'd probably better get a new wrap in case the evening got too chilly.

All of this happened the morning of the wedding, even though I had known about the event for months. Here I was, rushing around my apartment and even considering a quick shopping trip for new earrings and a wrap. It took a few moments for the reality to finally sink in, that no matter what I chose to wear, I would look great. After all, we were going to the wedding to celebrate the bride and groom on their big day. It was really about them, not us.

Oh, if you're wondering what I decided to wear—I wore my black mermaid gown, coordinating jewelry, wrap, and purse—all from my closet. Which pair of shoes did I choose? It was the three-inch blinged-out heels, which I later kicked off to dance. That evening, as I headed out the door, I knew I was going to have a great time. Looking back, what was worth remembering was the fun we had, not so much what we wore. The last-minute worry about what to wear only fed my anxiety and made me lose time that day—time and energy I could have put to better use.

Stay Healthy: Harness the Power of Meditation

"Silence is golden," my teachers used to say to us kids when we became too chatty in class. That line holds true when I think of meditation. More than "quiet time," meditation is a powerful way to bring a sense of calm, relaxation, and balance to your daily life.

Meditation is a practice that has been around for thousands of years. It generally refers to a practice of calming and recharging the mind and body, and it comes in different forms. Over the years, studies have looked at the effects of meditation on health.

For instance, researchers at Harvard University's Mind/Body Medical Institute found that meditation increases brain-wave activity, enhances intuition, improves concentration, and relieves some aches and pains.[7] It's not surprising that prominent companies like Deutsche Bank, AOL, Google, Time Warner, Nike, Apple, and others have realized the positive mental health benefits of meditation to the extent that they provide their employees spaces and classes for meditation.

A good place to start practicing meditation is with peaceful visualization. This involves taking your mind off its present business and focusing on calming images to help you turn tension into relaxation.

Your Daily Meditation Routine

1. Find a quiet, comfortable place.

2. Sit upright on a chair with your legs together, feet flat on the floor. You may also sit on the

---

7   Susan McGreevey, "Eight weeks to a better brain," Harvard Gazette, January 21, 2011, accessed April 18, 2017, http://news.harvard.edu/gazette/story/2011/01/eight-weeks-to-a-better-brain/.

floor with your legs crossed, or just stretch them out in front of you on the floor. You may even lie flat on your back, arms by your side, palms turned upward.

3. The position of your hands can help you maintain posture and focus. Here are some options:

   □ Place your wrists on your knees and relax your arms. Using each hand, touch the tip of your index finger and thumb together, or touch the tip of your little finger and thumb together.

   □ Clasp your hands, palms together, and bring your hands to the center of your chest, as you would during a prayer.

4. Close your eyes to block out any visual distractions. Block out all outside noises and commotions: radio, TV, people talking, traffic sounds. If possible, play soft, meditative sounds or music to help create the atmosphere for meditation.

5. Take a few deep breaths, then breathe naturally, focusing on your breath.

6. Picture a place that reminds you of something pleasant and then use your senses to "visualize" the scene. If it's a beach, hear the waves swooshing as they wash up on the shore. In a park, hear the birds chirping. In a

field of flowers, picture the colors and inhale the fragrances.

7. As you practice, naturally you'll find your mind wandering. When that happens, let those thoughts float by and bring yourself back to your original thought.

Whatever form mediation takes for you, invest the time and just be still. Live in and become absorbed in the moment. Remember in chapter 1 when I realized that I had spent my entire Saturday morning rushing around? Just when I began to feel accomplished, it occurred to me that I hadn't enjoyed the gift of a *free* morning. I attempted to do so many things that I thought needed to be done on schedule. Instead, I could have savored the natural rhythm of the day. Savoring a day's rhythm is something you can do at any time by pausing and meditating.

If you find yourself getting off on the wrong foot in the morning, meditation can help you get back on the right foot. If you are hurrying and having one of those mornings where you break the coffee mug, burn the toast, and put on the wrong shoes, you can still take a moment or two to pause, breathe, and find your center before heading out the door.

Many people with a meditation routine have the luxury of being able to be still for twenty minutes or more. But meditation is a skill that takes discipline. It will take time to build up to even ten minutes of undistracted focus. When distractions happen, just return your mind to your breathing. You will find that over time your thoughts will become more organized, and fresh ideas will flow in. Something that was difficult to grasp may even become clear. Keep paper and pen nearby when you meditate so that you can jot down ideas when they float by in your thoughts.

The trick is to keep practicing. Eventually it will be easy to do a ten-minute meditation. Remember, meditation can help reduce stress and quiet your spirit. A few moments alone in silence can help frame a good day, and help you stay healthy.

Do Meditative Breathing

Breathing exercises can help to relieve your body's natural reaction to stress. Meditative breathing fills the cells in your body with a fresh supply of oxygen, helping to reduce tension and lower blood pressure. Ultimately it helps to create balance and keep you calm and connected to your body. To begin, sit comfortably in a meditative pose and close your eyes, legs crossed and spine straight. If you are sitting on a chair, rest your feet flat on the ground. Focus on your breathing as you feel the sensations in your body come and go. Focus on how your breath feels as you inhale and exhale. Feel the rise and fall of your chest. Breathing deeply increases the supply of oxygen to your brain, and stimulates the part of the nervous system that helps to slow your heart rate and create a state of serenity.

Do Walking Meditation

Although meditation is often considered an exercise that involves sitting in place and gaining a sense of calm, it's also possible to meditate while you move—known as walking meditation.

Walking meditation is still about connecting to your body, focusing on your breathing, and being silent. It involves inhaling and exhaling as you put one foot in front of the other. It can be done indoors or out, but walking outdoors gives you a chance to connect with nature.

Choose a time of the day when you can walk uninterrupted for ten to thirty minutes. Wear comfortable shoes. Take a few deep breaths before you start, and become aware of your body. Walk at a slow, relaxed pace. Focus on your rhythm as you walk. Focus on your heel-to-toe motion as you alternate left and right feet. Pay attention to the sensations in your feet, ankles, legs, knees, thighs, hips, pelvis, abdomen, chest, back, shoulders, neck, and head. If you are outdoors, notice nature around you—trees, plants, birds. Again, remember to bring your thoughts back if they begin to wander.

chapter four takeaway

Begin your day with a peaceful morning routine. Use meditation to bring calm, relaxation, and balance to your life. Breathing is the key to successful meditation. As you breathe, focus your attention on the effect it has on your senses—make each thought, emotion, sound, and sensation that enters your mind envelope you.

An Exercise to Embrace Your Best Self

4-7-8 Breathing Stress Buster

Whenever you feel stress, this 4-7-8 Breathing Stress Buster exercise can help you quickly regain a sense of tranquility.

- Inhale through your nose with your mouth closed for a count of **four**.

- Hold your breath for a count of **seven**.

- Exhale through your mouth for a count of **eight**.

- Repeat this three times.

Use this exercise as often as you feel the need.

part two

Your Best Body

chapter five

Beauty Beyond Fifty

You can be beautiful at any age. However, we live in a society that influences us to fix things about ourselves. We are inundated with media and ads that scream, "You need to reverse the signs of aging to look more beautiful!" As a result, many of us end up with cabinets brimming with anti-aging products, potions, and makeup. We often struggle to resist the temptation to buy more. That's what happened to Brandy, a recruiter for a well-known tech company.

For her sixtieth birthday, Brandy received a spa day as a gift from her friends at work. The gift was a luxurious ninety-minute, full-body aromatherapy massage and a sixty-minute, anti-aging facial that promised to brighten her complexion and hydrate her skin. After an invigorating facial and massage, her facialist met her at the checkout counter with a slew of products—shea butter moisturizer, eye serum, anti-aging wrinkle cream, and Moroccan oil—some of the products used in her facial treatment. Brandy couldn't resist the temptation to buy the products. After all, she felt like a million bucks after her spa treatment. But the truth was, those specially formulated products would likely end up among her already brimming and expensive collection of anti-aging serums, moisturizers, night creams, day creams, blushes, eye pencils, mascara, eyelash enhancer, foundation, body butters, and hair care remedies.

Brandy is not alone in her cosmetic buying habits. According to research by Mint.com, the average woman spends as much as $15,000 on makeup in her lifetime. Not surprising, four in five women wear makeup, and 50 percent believe that makeup gives them a leg up at work and makes them feel in control.[8]

At age fifty and beyond, you have earned the right to be comfortable in your own skin. You see beauty differently at your age, and you know that age does not define beauty because beauty truly comes from within.

The issue isn't only the definition of "beauty." It is also the clever and persuasive ad industry that equates beauty with youth. Being flooded with ads for tighter, wrinkle-free skin, vanishing cellulite, and thick, voluminous hair—can naturally impact how a woman feels about herself. Beauty ads are designed to appeal psychologically to a woman's emotions and affect how she views herself. Comparing herself to the images shown can cause a woman to lower her self-esteem. The ads for beauty-enhancing products promise women believable, dramatic results, and these ads are very effective—women

---

8   Ross Crooks, "Splurge vs. save: Which beauty products are worth the extra cost?" Mint.com, April 11, 2013, accessed April 18, 2017, https://blog.mint.com/consumer-iq/splurge-vs-save-which-beauty-products-are-worth-the-extra-cost-0413/?display=wide.

spend billions of dollars on beauty products as shortcuts to being fabulous and healthy.

Frankly, there are products on the market that do make a woman look and feel good. It feels good to apply a fragrant facial cream that makes your skin feel softer and look more radiant. It feels good to look in the mirror and see healthy looking, more manageable hair after using a certain shampoo. It feels good to put on shapewear that delivers the smooth, flat appearance you love when you wear a close-fitting dress.

Being flooded with ads for tighter, wrinkle-free skin, vanishing cellulite, and thick, voluminous hair—can naturally impact how a woman feels about herself.

But, as women age, it can be difficult to identify with ads featuring much younger women. Many women do not see themselves reflected in ads, movies, or TV. Those ads featuring middle-aged women are rarely about beauty; instead they may promote medications, supplements, or disposable undies that offer extra protection for an overactive bladder.

A recent Dove Global Beauty and Confidence study that interviewed over 10,500 women and girls across thirteen countries, showed that 60 percent of women believe they need to meet certain beauty standards. The good news is that 83 percent of the women said they want to look their personal best rather than follow someone else's definition of beauty.[9]

---

9   "New Dove research finds beauty pressures up, and women and girls calling for change," PRNewswire, June 21, 2016, https://www.prnewswire.com/news-releases/new-dove-research-finds-beauty-pressures-up-and-women-and-girls-calling-for-change-583743391.html.

So, it's time to redefine "beautiful"—to move the focus away from the commercialized emphasis on youthfulness and back to being fabulous and healthy in mind, body, and spirit. It's time to love the skin you live in. Beauty is no longer reserved for the young, wrinkle-free woman with voluminous hair. Today, gray hair, plus sizes, and other previously perceived imperfections are perfectly acceptable. Beauty is about being comfortable in your own skin. Beauty is your reality—and not an unrealistic, heavily edited magazine photo spread. Beauty is ageless.

> **It's time to redefine "beautiful"—to move the focus away from the commercialized emphasis on youthfulness and back to being fabulous and healthy in mind, body, and spirit.**

In her book, *Prime Time*, actress and former workout queen Jane Fonda writes, "Genes may predispose us to, say, heart disease or arthritis, but the right lifestyle and the right attitude may help us overcome these infirmities. I know older people who are disabled and even ill but who do not *feel* sick. They experience joy and vitality and, in my opinion, exemplify successful aging."[10]

You, too, should celebrate and embrace your own beauty at your age.

The truth is, every woman experiences changes that come with aging. So it may take a little tweaking from time to time to keep looking fabulous. But don't give up on beauty and health. Being your fabulous self is something wonderful, something extraordinary,

10   Jane Fonda, *Prime Time: Love, Health, Sex, Fitness, Friendship, Spirit; Making the Most of All of Your Life,* Random House, 2012.

something a little bit more than the usual. It's about being better than just okay—it's about being amazing inside and out. You can look and feel great about yourself no matter your age. These days, looking and feeling better is easier than before. I'll share more with you about how to improve how you feel about yourself in the chapters to come.

Be Fabulous: Find and Celebrate Your Personal Style

Your personal style can help you look and feel fabulous. Today, style cuts across all age groups; you can dress as fabulously at age sixty-five as you would have when you were thirty. Defining your personal style starts with understanding yourself: the image you want to convey, the statement you want to make, and the look that flatters you the most.

Although I enjoy fashion, I am not obsessed with it. I rarely plan what I am going to wear on a given day. Instead, I dress from the inside out. I dress the way I feel that day. I randomly choose what I want to wear, and in the end I'm usually happy with my decision. I feel great about myself without much fuss and preplanning. But if you are not the decisive type, it's better to decide on what to wear the night before. You might even plan your wardrobe for the entire week.

When it comes to updating your look, first recognize that there is a difference between fashion and style. Fashion is composed of trends that are sometimes short lived. Style, on the other hand, is expressing yourself through what you wear. Style is like your stamp—your own personal brand. The pieces you wear can create the impression that you are your own person. What you wear, how you look, is really an extension of who you are—your personality and your individuality. It's a look that is exclusively yours. That's your personal style.

You don't need to spend a lot to create a personal style that spells *quality*. With a few wise decisions, you can find clothes that will always be in style. There are foundation pieces that you can always accessorize and dress up or down. Then you can add what I call *investment pieces* to your collection—those special-occasion pieces that cost a bit more but won't go out of style anytime soon.

> **What you wear, how you look, is really an extension of who you are—your personality and your individuality. It's a look that is exclusively yours.**

Purge Your Closet

Before you go shopping to add other pieces and create your personal style, you need to get a full picture of what you already have. Now is the perfect time for a closet purge. Chances are you'll find things you forgot you had, some outdated, some you've held on to for too long, and some that no longer reflect who you are.

A closet purge was the best starting point for fashionista, Candy. She knew her closets were bursting at the seams, overflowing with clothes, hats, shoes, and her favorite thing—handbags. Too overwhelmed to take on the task by herself, she invited two friends over for what she called a "closet clean-out and a glass of chardonnay." Between sips of chardonnay, it didn't take them long to find things Candy hadn't worn in years and wouldn't dare wear now. They found clothes that no longer fit and dresses, sweaters, and handbags still bearing their original price tags. When it was all over, Candy had well-organized, less-crowded closets. From the piles of things she no longer needed, she took a few pieces to a consignment store and donated the rest to the neighborhood Goodwill.

Begin your own closet cleanup.

1. Pull everything out of your closets and drawers.

2. Organize each item in groups by season (spring/summer, fall/winter). That includes scarves, hats, bags, belts, and shoes. Sorting may take a few days, so focus on one group of clothing each day.

3. Organize the items in batches by color, type of clothing, and/or style. For example, it could be all sweaters, or all professional, casual, or dressy clothes. Organize shoes by either color or casual style vs. dressy—flats, pumps, or sandals.

4. With each batch of clothes, create three piles: "yes," "no," and "maybe." Place the items you want to keep in the "yes" pile, those you want to donate or give away in the "no" pile, and anything you have difficulty deciding about in the "maybe" pile.

5. Then go through the "maybe" pile and try the items on. Look in the mirror and decide whether it still fits and looks good on you. Those items that have seen better days should go in the "no" pile.

6. Once everything is sorted, put the items in the "yes" pile back in your closet and drawers and organize them by category and color. For example, hang the dresses together by color and by occasion—day, evening, or casual wear.

Now make a shopping list, just like you would for groceries. Think about the style gaps you need to fill. What's missing? What do you need to go with things you already have? What are must haves? What pieces will perk up your look?

Be a Savvy Shopper

The fact that style cuts across all age groups is the reason my daughter is my favorite shopping buddy. Get a shopping buddy who can help you select classic pieces that are affordable and that fit and flatter you.

Do a little research before you shop to see what's trending. You can get inspiration from image consultants' websites or women's magazines. However, don't be a slave to fashion and fall for trends that don't make sense to you.

Select classic pieces that are affordable and that fit and flatter you.

As fashion guru Tim Gunn, consultant to TV's *Project Runway* and the former chair of the fashion design department at New York's Parsons School of Design says, "Refresh your style through good quality, comfortable undergarments, and figure-flattering sizes, fabrics, and colors."

So refresh your style and try new pieces and colors to see what works. Start with a few wardrobe staples, like a basic black pantsuit and black blazer, a little black dress and black skirt, black pants and a cropped jacket, black and white Ts, a crisp white shirt and jeans. These are foundational pieces that you can use to build a solid but flexible wardrobe. Freshen these up with other pieces that match your personality. My friend Barbara likes to pair jeans with vintage blouses. She keeps a list of style combinations that worked for her in the past, especially those that earned her compliments.

Now that you've established your wardrobe essentials, build your accessories around them. Accessories are versatile and can be paired with something unexpected to reflect your personal style. Scarves are especially fun; they give you room to experiment and bring in splashes of color whenever you need it. Belts always seem to be in fashion, and necklaces—long or short, single or layered—are a great way to pull your look together.

Showcase your favorite features and accentuate them without overdoing it. Look at yourself in the mirror, and honestly assess your assets. If you have great shoulders and arms, show them off. If you have a great butt, by all means dress to show it off. If your legs are shapely, wear more dresses and skirts. Dress for your body shape. If you have a slim waist, wear clothes or belts that cinch it in. Whether you're slim, petite, curvy, or plus size, you have assets that you should celebrate.

Don't worry about the old rules of avoiding white after Labor Day or wearing only black if you are full-figured. Whatever your age and body type, wear clothes that fit well. Well-fitting clothes will complement your body, so dress for your body type and make it size appropriate. In most cases, oversized clothes visually add pounds, making you look bigger than you really are. Of course, wear what's comfortable, but if you are working on updating your look and you are full-figured, don't let baggy clothes be your personal style.

Keeping your look simple, fresh, fun, and colorful speaks volumes about the inner you. After all, dressing fabulously is more about reflecting outward how you feel on the inside. Small changes don't have to cost a bundle, and can make the difference in how you look and feel. Once you know what works for you and what looks best on your body type, the rest is easy.

Finding your personal style means knowing what works and being bold about it. It means loving the way you look in what you wear and *owning it*. It's your signature, your brand. Finding your personal style will help improve your self-confidence and the way others see you.

Reinvent Your Look

Having a great wardrobe is a good way to start making yourself look and feel good. But there are other ways to update your look.

Admittedly, some women get stuck and are afraid to let go—they have held on to their *look* for far too long. Same hair, same makeup, same style. That was the look they had when they felt the most youthful and attractive. If this is you, it's time to climb out of the time capsule and get a makeover—small changes can shed years and make a world of difference in your appearance.

These days, there are websites, blogs, and videos for just about everything, from applying makeup, creating beautiful brows, and changing hairstyles to mixing and matching clothes for a perfect look.

Hair is the quickest and most noticeable change a woman can make. A change in your hairstyle or color can make a big difference in how you feel about yourself. That's all it took for Jill, a sixty-year-old accounting clerk. When Jill sashayed into the room at her company's holiday party, her friends barely recognized her. She had changed her hair color from auburn to dark brown; the result was stunning. The change complemented her skin color and brought out the color of her brown eyes. She looked happy and had a warm glow about her. Jill felt the immediate emotional impact—she felt more self-confident as she made her way through the party.

A new hairstyle, color, cut, or a more natural look can make a world of difference in your appearance. Some women hang onto their long hair forever, and there are those who can pull off having long hair at any age. But

Hair is the quickest and most noticeable change a woman can make. A change in your hairstyle or color can make a big difference in how you feel about yourself.

now could be the time to take a risk and experiment—bobs, bangs, braids, natural, messy, layered, extensions, wigs, or a new color are among the many options these days. Go with a cut that accents your face and a color that makes you stand out. The results could be stunning. Whatever changes you decide on for your hair, make it one that is easy to style and care for.

Stay Healthy: Turn Back the Clock with Good Skin Care

We know that beauty *isn't* only skin deep, but that doesn't mean you can ignore your body's largest organ—your skin. It deserves plenty of attention if you are to keep it looking healthy.

Although the outer layer is what you see every day, your skin is actually made up of three layers: the epidermis, dermis, and subcutaneous fat. The *epidermis,* or outer layer, is part of your body's immune system. It makes new skin cells and melanin, which gives your skin its color. The *dermis,* or middle layer, contains sweat glands and oil glands to help keep your skin soft and smooth. This layer has hair follicles and nerve endings so that you can feel sensations like heat, cold, and pain, and it's in this layer that blood vessels remove waste from your skin and help keep your skin healthy. The *subcutaneous fat* (the third layer) attaches the dermis (middle layer) to your muscles and bones. This layer stores fat and helps keep your body temperature normal.[11]

Taking care of your skin means keeping it clean, protecting it from the sun, and nourishing it with a healthy diet. Some women are lucky to have "genes" that give them naturally flawless looking skin, but if your skin needs attention, there are steps you can take to let your radiance shine through every day.

Have a cleansing routine. Good skin care begins with proper cleansing. Cleansing removes dirt, unclogs pores, and sloughs off dead skin. A daily routine of cleaning your face with a good cleanser is first and foremost. Although the experience of washing your face and the sensation of splashing water all over it feels refreshing and

---

11 "The layers of your skin," American Academy of Dermatology, accessed April 18, 2017, https://www.aad.org/public/kids/skin/the-layers-of-your-skin.

exhilarating, facial cleansing towelettes are also effective. You can find a wide variety of facial cleansers and makeup removers in any health and beauty aisle. Some have gentle formulas that work for different skin types and sensitive eye areas. If you have problem areas—ultra-dry or extra oily facial skin—you may need specially formulated cleansers to take care of these problems.

> **Taking care of your skin means keeping it clean, protecting it from the sun, and nourishing it with a healthy diet.**

Cleansing and moisturizing suggestions

- **For dry skin**, use a mild, creamy, soap-free cleanser. Moisturize with a hydrating cream or lotion.

- **For oily skin**, use a cleanser with salicylic or alpha-hydroxy acid to get rid of any dead skin and unplug your pores. Moisturize with a light cream or lotion that won't block your pores.

- **For combination skin**, use an oil-free, foam cleanser with salicylic acid to help get rid of the excess oil without drying out your skin. Moisturize the same the way you would for oily skin.

- **For normal skin**, use a gentle, soap-free formula. Moisturize using a light non-comedogenic (non-pore blocking) formula.

Whatever you use, remember that over-cleansing is unnecessary and will rob your skin of its natural, healthy oils. So whatever your age or skin type, a gentle skin cleanser is always best.

Pamper yourself with a facial. A facial treatment is one way to pamper yourself and give your skin the extra hydration it needs. A facial treatment deep cleans, exfoliates, and tightens your skin. It opens up your pores and removes dirt and toxins. If you are adventurous and want to create your own concoction, you need go no further than your kitchen. Everything you need may be in your pantry or refrigerator. Avocado is not just for salads; a homemade avocado facial is chockfull of vitamins and natural oils that can help soften and hydrate your skin. Avocado can be combined with olive oil, egg whites, lemon juice, honey, and orange juice to create a noncommercial product that is free of chemicals.[12] If you have known allergies to specific fruits or vegetables, check with your doctor first before using them in a mask.

Exfoliate for a fresher look. Removing dead skin cells can help you look fresher and healthier. Exfoliating clears away old, dead cells from the surface of your skin, making the way for new cells to emerge. Exfoliating also helps even out your skin tone, unplug your pores, and reduce fine lines on your face.

It's best to exfoliate no more than once a week. Be careful not to over-scrub and irritate your skin. If you have skin problems like frequent outbreaks or acne, see a dermatologist. You may also consider microdermabrasion (a noninvasive treatment that sloughs off dead skin cells) with a dermatologist or a licensed skin care specialist.

Plump up your skin. Your cells love water, so drink up and plump up your skin from the inside out. Drink plenty of water to nourish tone and protect your skin. Ultimately, good hydrating helps to reduce premature wrinkles. Seal in the moisture by applying a moisturizing cream or lotion right after cleaning your skin while it

---

12   Denise Minger, "How to make an avocado facial mask," Livestrong.com, http://www.livestrong.com/article/95568-make-avocado-facial-mask/.

is still damp. Massage in the moisturizer for about fifteen seconds to help increase circulation. Sheet masks are great because the moisture won't evaporate. Nourishing your skin at night is important. Remember to moisturize the skin around your eyes and neck. The skin in these areas is especially thin and less oily so they are the first to show signs of aging.

Shun too much sun. Skin comes in a myriad of shades. Remember, melanin in the outer layer of your skin (the epidermis) is responsible for your skin color.[13] Your body makes more melanin when it is exposed to the sun. How much your body makes depends on your genes. The more melanin your skin makes, the darker your skin. Melanin gives you some protection against wrinkles, so people with darker skin tend to wrinkle much later in life.

Although melanin offers this natural protection against the sun's rays, everyone must protect their skin. The ultraviolet rays from the sun can trigger dark spots and premature wrinkles, and can even cause skin cancer.

To protect your skin from ultraviolet rays, choose a moisturizer that also contains sunscreen. Ideally, use a sunscreen that blocks long-wavelength ultraviolet light (UVA), which penetrates deep below the top layer of the skin. Your sunscreen should also block short-wavelength ultraviolet light (UVB), which causes sunburn on the surface of the skin. What's important to know is that UVA can age us, and UVB can burn us and even cause cancer. The bottom line: use a sunscreen that blocks both UVA and UVB rays.

Sunscreens have a sun protection factor (SPF) number that tells you how good the sunscreen is at blocking ultraviolet (UV) rays. The higher the number, the more protection it gives. Use a broad-spec-

---

13 "The layers of your skin," American Academy of Dermatology, accessed April 18, 2017, https://www.aad.org/public/kids/skin/the-layers-of-your-skin.

trum sunscreen with at least an SPF of thirty that blocks both UVA and UVB rays.[14] Clothing manufacturers are now making special UV-absorbing clothing labeled with an ultraviolet protection factor (UPF) rating. You can identify which clothes have this protection by looking for the seal on the labels. Wearing a wide-brimmed hat and UV-blocking sunglasses when you are out in the sun will also give you extra protection.

> **What's important to know is that UVA can age us, and UVB can burn us and even cause cancer.**

Eat, sleep, and exercise. As a registered, certified dietitian-nutritionist, I can't tell you the number of times women have asked me, "What should I do to make my skin, hair, and nails healthy?" My answer is always the same. I tell them, "Cleanse, moisturize, protect, and hydrate you skin, follow a healthy diet, and exercise."

For starters, drink lots of water to keep your skin hydrated and remove toxins from your body. Avoid stress, get enough sleep, and exercise regularly. This will reduce stress lines and increase blood flow to the surface of your skin, giving it a healthy look. Eat foods high in omega-3 fatty acids like salmon, walnuts, flaxseed, tofu, tuna, and mackerel. Eat fruits and vegetables that contain phytonutrients, anti-oxidant vitamins (A, E, and C), and minerals like zinc and iron for healthy skin, hair, and nails. In fact, researchers looking at nutrition and skin aging found that fruits and vegetables may be the healthiest and safest choices for maintaining a balanced diet and healthy-look-

---

14   "Skin cancer," Centers for Disease Control and Prevention, accessed April 18, 2017, https://www.cdc.gov/cancer/skin/basic_info/sun-safety.htm#sunscreen.

ing skin.[15] As much as possible, get these vitamins and minerals from foods, not supplements. In chapter 6 you will find more information on the best food sources for these nutrients.

Restore Your Radiance

If you've been wondering all along what happened to the radiance you once had, the answer is that the sun, stress, and pollution in the environment might have taken its toll. And although there is an abundance of anti-aging serums and wrinkle-reducing products on the market, slathering on too much won't necessarily bring you good results.

"Less is more" is a good rule to follow when it comes to makeup. Not everyone likes or needs makeup. Many women prefer to go all natural. But when used correctly, makeup can give a natural and flawless appearance. Even if you don't normally wear much makeup, a little might brighten a bare face. It can play up some features and play down others.

If you choose to wear makeup, try shades that match your skin tone. When in doubt, visit the makeup counter at any retail store and ask a makeup artist for help matching the right shades for your skin tone.

For best results, use good lighting when applying your makeup. Try using a primer as a base for your foundation; this allows it to go on smoother and last longer. Blend in foundation, concealer, eyeshadow, and blush well as you apply them at each step. Avoid applying eye, eyebrow, or lip makeup so heavily that it looks unnatural.

---

15 Silke Schagen et al., "Discovering the link between nutrition and skin aging," *Dermato Endocrinology* 4, no. 3 (July 2012): 298-307, accessed April 18, 2017, on U.S. National Library of Medicine, National Institutes of Health, https://www. ncbi.nlm.nih.gov/pmc/articles/PMC3583891/.

Don't fret if your eyebrows are growing thin and the natural color is fading. You can bring some definition back using a brow corrector or with a few feather-like strokes of a brow pencil for a natural look. Another alternative is microblading, a technique that uses a special pen to draw precise, hair-like strokes to make the perfect look-alike brows. If you wear mascara to make your lashes stand out, consider a waterproof variety to prevent smudging. If you use eyeliner to help define and brighten your eyes, keep it soft and subtle.

Sometimes a concealer can be your best friend, especially if you get dark under-eye circles or need coverage for minor skin discoloration. For a more natural look, apply it lightly and blend it evenly so that it looks natural and to avoid "raccoon eyes."

It's never too late to restore your radiance. You're going to be seen wherever you go, so why not be seen in your best light?

Win with a Smile

One of the best ways to peel back the years is having a winning smile. Research shows that the appearance of your teeth can affect your self-confidence and happiness. Of course, a great smile means clean, bright, and healthy teeth. If you have yellow or brown stains caused by coffee, tea, wine, or other foods, an easy fix is to have your dentist whiten your teeth. If you are the do-it-yourself type, there are a number of whitening and bleaching options in the health and beauty section of your local supermarket or pharmacy. Twice-a-year visits to the dentist will pay big dividends when it comes to having a winning smile.

chapter five takeaway

It's never too late to refresh your style, restore your radiance, and reinvent your look.

With good skin care, diet, exercise, and rest, you can tap into your fountain of youth and look your best. Appreciate your beauty, take the time to enhance it and preserve it. Love the older skin that you live in—you've earned that right.

An Exercise to Embrace Your Best Self

Your Best Body Checklist

Take this health checklist to see where you are today.

1. I feel _____ most days.

2. When I look in the mirror I feel _____.

3. When I wake up in the morning, I first spend time doing this: _____.

4. I exercise _____time(s) a week.

5. I eat _____ meal(s) a day.

6. I eat _____serving(s) of fruits a day.

7. I eat _____ serving(s) of vegetables a day.

8. I eat _____ serving(s) of whole grains a day.

9. I feel pain in _____ of my body.

10. I have seen a doctor to discuss my health issues.
    Yes_____ No_____

11. I connect with friends and/or family members _____ time(s) a week.

12. I _____ for recreation _____ time(s) a week/month.

How did you do with this checklist?_____

Did it show you that you have some work to do?

_____

Did it show that you need to:

Eat more healthy foods? _____

Visit your doctor? _____

Connect with others? _____

Renew your self-confidence? _____

chapter six

Nutrition—Eat for Life

Early in my career I worked in the outpatient clinic of a large municipal New York hospital. There I met many people with serious health issues such as diabetes, heart disease, high blood pressure, cancer, and obesity. Most of them did not know what foods to eat to improve their health.

One day during one of my weight reduction sessions, Mindy, a regular member of the group, looked at me and laughed out loud after I told them that half a cup of rice was one serving. In Mindy's culture, rice was a staple food. It was normal for her to eat one cup or more at lunch and dinner.

Then there was Ali, who I met a few weeks after she was diagnosed with diabetes. She was confused about what foods to eat to get her blood sugar under control. She was bombarded with advice from friends, which often conflicted with the advice she received from her doctor.

These days, women are eager for information about healthy eating, weight loss, fitness, food allergies, probiotics, prebiotics, vegetarianism, and gluten-free, organic, antibiotic-free, and hormone-free foods. Mostly, they're looking to make healthy lifestyle changes. They want to eat foods to prevent and control disease.

According to a nutrition trends survey by the Academy of Nutrition and Dietetics, although people were less satisfied with the way they ate, their main reason for not eating "healthfully" was their longtime, well-established eating habits. Many said they did not know or understand the dietary guidelines or exactly what foods make up *healthy eating*.

Healthy aging starts with you—it does not happen overnight.

Healthy aging starts with you—it does not happen overnight. It's like putting money into a savings account and waiting for it to give you a return. Healthy eating is one of the cornerstones of healthy aging. Healthy eating can add years to your life. It can prevent or even reverse chronic diseases like obesity, heart disease, high cholesterol, and high blood pressure.

Healthy eating means your diet must include whole foods—foods in their original form. A dietary supplement may give you short-term relief if you are deficient in a certain nutrient. For example, if your calcium levels are low, your doctor may prescribe a calcium supplement and suggest you eat plenty of calcium-rich foods. But your body is designed to get the most nutrition benefits from whole foods, not just from supplements or processed foods. Whole foods are packed with antioxidant vitamins, minerals, and phytonutrients (plant-based nutrients) that protect your body from *free radicals*. These free radicals form as a result of certain natural processes occurring in your body and from influences from the environment—your diet, stress level, smoking and drinking habits, exercise regimen, inflammation, drug use, exposure to sunlight, and pollution. Free radicals can damage the cells in your body and make you more susceptible to disease and aging if they are not gobbled up by antioxidants.[16]

Be Healthy, Reshape Your Plate

Now that you know you should eat "healthfully," how will you do it? You start by reshaping your plate. Take a look at a plate with the foods you normally eat. Is the plate loaded with foods that are salty, high in calories, sugar, and fat? Is the plate skimpy on fruits and vegetables? If the answer to either of these questions is "yes," then it's time to reshape your plate. At least two-thirds of your plate should be made up of plant-based foods like vegetables, fruits, whole grains, and beans. The remaining one-third can come from animal foods like meat, poultry, seafood, and dairy products. Think of meat as a condiment, not the main focus of your meal. This means meat should only be a small portion—no more than three ounces—and just enough to complement the rest of the food on your plate.

Keep a Food Journal

As you begin working on reshaping your plate, create an eating pattern that best meets your personal nutritional needs. Start with the foods you like and gradually add new ones. A food journal will give you a good picture of your eating patterns and the types of foods

---

16   V. Lobo et al., "Free radicals, antioxidants and functional foods: Impact on human health," *Pharmacognosy Review* 4, no. 8 (July-December 2010): 118-126, accessed June 1, 2017, on U.S. National Library of Medicine, National Institutes of Health, www.ncbi.nlm.nih.gov/pmc/articles/PMC3249911/.

you eat. It will also help you pinpoint whether you are eating emotionally, and which habits you need to break.

There are a number of smartphone apps that you can use to keep a digital food journal, or you can keep a written journal using the sample journal provided below. If you're using a written journal, be sure to include the day of the week, the date, your meals, and the time of day you have your meals.

For two weeks, list everything you eat and drink, including snacks and munchies. Be specific and describe the food (e.g., is the bread white or whole grain bread?), the amounts (e.g., one cup, two slices), and how the food was prepared (e.g., fried, baked, or steamed). Include beverages (tea, coffee, juices, smoothies, shakes, liquor, and water) as well as condiments (butter, sugar, and dressings). Include where you were when you ate (restaurant, home), what you were doing (with friends, alone), and how you felt when you were eating (happy, sad). The journal helps you to see if you are eating because you feel hungry or because you are happy, bored, stressed, depressed, angry, or fatigued.

Your Food Journal

DAY OF THE WEEK: _____ **DATE:** _____

MEAL	TIME	PLACE AND ACTIVITY	FOOD OR BEVERAGE, HOW IT WAS PREPARED	AMOUNT	FEELINGS BEFORE EATING
BREAKFAST					
LUNCH					
DINNER					
SNACK					

Chances are, when you're in your fifties and beyond, you have a less active, more sedentary lifestyle. If you work, your work may involve sitting at a desk. If this is true, you will need fewer calories than you did in your twenties.

So how much food should you eat to stay healthy? It all comes down to quality. Better quality food means food with the essential nutrients you need, not empty calories that won't do your body any favors.

This brings me to the topic of subconscious or mindless eating. According to Brian Wansink, a food psychologist at Cornell University, mindless eating is "about reengineering your environment so that you can eat what you want without guilt and without gaining weight. It's about reengineering your food life so that it is enjoyable and mindful."[17] Health experts today suggest that we should eat only when we're hungry, and stop when we're full. But how many times have you gone to the movie theater and, before you know it, you've eaten an entire bucket of popcorn—a bucket so full that at first you thought you could never finish it? If your mind is occupied with a movie while eating, your brain is likely to miss the signal telling you to stop when you're full.

To overcome mindless eating, slow down and pay attention to the tastes, smells, and textures of your food. Whenever possible, avoid serving food family style, as this will undoubtedly entice you to

> **To overcome mindless eating, slow down and pay attention to the tastes, smells, and textures of your food.**

---

17   Hale, Jamie, "Mindless Eating," PsychCentral, book review accessed June 1, 2017, https://psychcentral.com/lib/mindless-eating/.

reach for more. Use a smaller plate and fill it only once. In the end, you will eat less.

When you are reshaping your plate and learning to eat healthfully, there are a number of "do"s and "don't"s to keep in mind.

Eat Less of These

Bad fats – Skip it, skim it, or trim it. *Bad fats* include industrially made trans fats and saturated fats. *Trans fats* raise the level of *bad* low-density lipoprotein (LDL) cholesterol and lower the level of *good* high-density lipoprotein (HDL) cholesterol in your blood. High LDL and low HDL can increase the risk of heart disease, stroke, diabetes, and other chronic health conditions.

Trans fats were once prevalent in many commercially prepared foods, but recent government regulations now require food companies to remove or cut back on trans fats in foods and put the amount of trans fat on the nutrition facts labels. *Saturated fats* are found in animal foods like meats, chicken, whole milk, whole-milk dairy foods, and coconut oil. Saturated fats can cause your total cholesterol and LDL cholesterol to go up. This can block the arteries in your heart and elsewhere in your body and cause a heart attack.

Sugar – Resist the urge to eat sugary foods and drink sugary beverages. Sodas, fruit punches, energy drinks, and sports drinks often contain some form of refined sugar. Read the label; cane sugar, high-fructose corn syrup, corn syrup, agave nectar, and dextrose are forms of sugar that have empty calories and have little or no nutritional benefit. What's more, research shows that sugary foods increase the risk of weight gain, diabetes, and heart disease.

Refined grains – Pass on refined grains. Refined grains include white rice, white flour, and products made with white flour, such as some breads, crackers, desserts, pastries, and breakfast cereals. Refined grains are milled to give them a finer texture and to keep them fresh longer, but milling strips away the bran and germ. Although refined grain products are enriched or fortified with the vitamins and minerals lost during this process, they are still missing key nutrients when compared to whole grains.

Alcohol – If you drink at all, drink only in moderation. For women, that means no more than one drink per day and for men no more than two. A standard drink is twelve ounces of beer, one and a half ounces of distilled spirits, or five ounces of wine—they all have the same amount of alcohol. According to the American Cancer Society, heavy alcohol drinking can cause health problems, including increasing your risk of cancer.[18]

Salt – Shake the salt habit. Use less salt. When you cook, don't add salt. Remove the salt shaker from the table, and don't add salt to food at the table before you eat. Use flavor enhancers like vibrant herbs and spices to wake up the natural flavor of foods.

Many foods are notoriously high in salt, so cut the amount of salt in your diet by eating less salty snacks and processed meats like cold cuts, hot dogs, and sausages. A salt substitute may be a good alternative, but talk with your health professional first because salt substitutes are high in potassium and may cause your potassium levels to go up.

---

18 "Alcohol Use and Cancer," The American Cancer Society, cancer.org, (April 2017): https://www.cancer.org/cancer/cancer-causes/diet-physical-activity/alcohol-use-and-cancer.html.

Wake Up Flavors with Spices

- **Basil:** lamb, lean ground meats, stews, salads, soups, sauces, seafood

- **Bay leaves:** lean meats, stews, poultry, soups, tomatoes

- **Chopped chives:** salads, sauces, soups, lean meat dishes, vegetables

- **Vinegar:** salads, vegetables, sauces, seafood

- **Curry:** lean meats (especially lamb), veal, chicken, seafood, tomatoes, tomato soup

- **Dill:** seafood sauces, soups, tomatoes, cabbage, carrots, cauliflower, green beans, cucumbers, potatoes, salads, macaroni, lean beef, lamb, chicken, seafood

- **Fresh garlic or garlic powder (not garlic salt):** lean meats, seafood, soups, salads, vegetables, tomatoes, potatoes

- **Fresh onion or onion powder** (not onion salt): lean meats, stews, seafood, vegetables, salads, soups

- **Ginger:** chicken, lean meats, seafood

- **Lemon:** lean meats, seafood, chicken, turkey, salads, vegetables

- **Mustard (dry):** lean meats, chicken, seafood, salads, asparagus, broccoli, Brussels sprouts, cabbage, sauces

- **Paprika:** lean meats, seafood, soups, salads, sauces, vegetables
- **Parsley:** lean meats, seafood, soups, salads, sauces, vegetables

---

Eat More of These

Fruits and vegetables – Fill half your plate with fruits and vegetables. They are packed with fiber, vitamins A and C, calcium, folate, potassium, and a host of plant nutrients. Fruits and vegetables have little or no fat and are low in calories. They also have no cholesterol. Eating lots of fruits and vegetables can help reduce your cancer risk. The American Cancer Society recommends eating at least two and a half cups of these every day.[19] Eat a variety of fruits and vegetables, especially those that are brightly colored.

Legumes – Legumes are healthy substitutes for animal protein. They include peas, beans, and lentils. The most versatile and nutritious legumes are chick peas, black-eyed peas, and kidney, fava, lima, black, and edamame (green soy) beans. Legumes are generally low in fat, contain no cholesterol, and are high in fiber, folate, potassium, iron, zinc, B vitamins, and magnesium. Although legumes do not have all of the essential amino acids (smaller units of protein), they are great in salads, stews, soups, and casseroles.

---

19 "It's Easy to Add Fruits and Vegetables to Your Diet," The American Cancer Society, cancer.org, (October 2013): https://www.cancer.org/healthy/eat-healthy-get-active/eat-healthy/add-fruits-and-veggies-to-your-diet.html.

Whole grains – Whole grains are nature's way of serving up *good carbs*. At least half of all the grains in your diet should be whole grains. As the name suggests, "whole grains" means the entire grain kernel—the bran, germ, and endosperm are intact. Some examples of whole grains are whole wheat flour, bulgur, oats, bran, whole cornmeal, brown and black rice, farro, quinoa, and wheat berry. These are rich in vitamins B and E, calcium, zinc, and iron. A big bonus is that they are packed with fiber and complex (unrefined) carbohydrates (good carbs). These make you feel full quickly, help to control your blood sugar levels, and keep your bowels healthy.

> **Whole grains are nature's way of serving up *good carbs*.**

Protein foods – Healthy proteins include lean meat, chicken, turkey, eggs, beans, peas, lentils, soy products, and unsalted nuts and seeds. Although animal protein provides the essential amino acids your body needs, the leaner the better. Leaner meats are healthy because they have less saturated fat (bad fat) and less fat overall. Studies now show that eating healthy proteins like fish, chicken, beans, or nuts in place of red meat and processed meats like deli meats can help to lower the risk of certain diseases. For example, eating a lot of red meats and processed meats can increase the risk of colon cancer. Women, especially, can reduce their risk of heart disease significantly by swapping red meats and processed meats for leaner proteins in their meals.[20]

---

20 "Recommendations for cancer prevention," American Institute for Cancer Research, accessed June 1, 2017, http://www.aicr.org/reduce-your-cancer-risk/recommendations-for-cancer-prevention/recommendations_05_red_meat.html.

Good fats – During the 1960s, a study of seven countries in the Mediterranean showed that most of the people in Greece and other parts of the Mediterranean lived long lives. What was astounding was that few of these people had heart disease and certain cancers even though they ate high-fat diets. As it turned out, their diets also included lots of fruits, vegetables, whole grain cereals, nuts, legumes, fish, olive oil, and moderate amounts of chicken and turkey—but only small amounts of red meats.[21] Today this is known as the Mediterranean diet, and it is highly recommended by health experts as a healthy way to eat.

Honestly, we all need some fat for energy and cell membranes and to protect nerves, help muscles move, and improve how we absorb certain vitamins and minerals. However, you should focus on getting more of the *good fats*. Good fats include monounsaturated fats, polyunsaturated fats, and omega-3 and omega-6 fatty acids. *Monounsaturated fats* are plentiful in olive oil, peanut oil, canola oil, avocados, most nuts, and safflower and sunflower oils. *Polyunsaturated fats* are plentiful in vegetable oils like corn, sunflower, and safflower oils. The best sources of *omega-3* are flaxseeds, walnuts, canola oil, un-hydrogenated soybean oil, and fatty fish like salmon, mackerel, and sardines. The best sources of

> **The good fats help to lower the levels of the *bad* LDL cholesterol and triglycerides (types of fats in our bloodstream), and in so doing help prevent heart disease and stroke.**

---

21   Anastasios Dontas et al., "Mediterranean diet and prevention of coronary heart disease in the elderly," *Clinical Interventions in Aging* 2, no. 1 (March 2007): 109-115, accessed June 1, 2017, on U.S. National Library of Medicine, National Institutes of Health, https://www.ncbi.nlm.nih.gov/pmc/articles/PMC2684076/.

omega-6 are walnut oil and vegetable oils like corn, sunflower, safflower, and soybean. The good fats help to lower the levels of the *bad* LDL cholesterol and triglycerides (types of fats in our bloodstream), and in so doing help prevent heart disease and stroke.

Fluids – Don't wait until you feel thirsty to hydrate. Water makes up about 60 percent of your body, so you need it to survive, and you need plenty of it to keep organs like your brain and heart functioning at peak performance. You need water for healthy digestion, skin, muscles, and joints and to keep your body temperature normal. Water carries nutrients to your cells and flushes out toxins (poisons) and wastes from your body.

To stay refreshed and hydrated every day, drink about eight to twelve eight-ounce glasses of water every day. Jumpstart your day and flush your digestive system after a long night's sleep by drinking a glass of water spiked with lemon juice. If plain water is too bland, add some zest with teas or flavored waters. Make your own flavored waters by adding any combination of lemon, orange, lime, grapefruit, kiwi, ginger, watermelon, cucumbers, strawberries, apples, and pineapple. The bottom line is keep water handy, especially during hot weather and when you work out.

Calcium – Calcium and vitamin D—the sunshine vitamin—are important for women in preventing osteoporosis (brittle and fragile bones) and keeping your bones healthy. Health experts suggest that if you are over fifty, you need 1,200 mg of calcium every day. Remember, food is your best source for calcium. Include foods in your diet like low-fat and nonfat milk, yogurt, cheese, canned fish (with soft bones) like salmon and sardines, and vegetables like broccoli, soybeans, and dark-green leafy greens like kale, collards, and spinach. Check the labels of juices, breakfast cereals, milk, and breads to find those with added calcium.

Read Labels

One way to rein in unhealthy eating habits is to understand food labeling. Once in a while you may crave a treat, but get into the habit of checking food labels for the nutrients and ingredients in a single serving. One bag of your favorite snack could contain as many as four servings—you could unwittingly overindulge and eat all four servings at once.

Take a close look at the ingredients on the label. The main ingredient is listed first, followed by the ingredients that are included in smaller amounts. For instance, a bag of potato chips may list the ingredients as "potatoes, sunflower oil, and salt," while a bag of Tostitos may read, "whole white corn, vegetable oil (corn, soybean, canola, and/or sunflower oil), and salt."

The nutrition facts label for packaged foods makes it easier for you to find out which foods are more healthful. This sample label shows things to look for in a food product.[22]

---

22 "The New and Improved Nutrition Facts Label–Key Changes," US Food and Drug Administration, June 2017, https://www.fda.gov/downloads/food/ingredientspackaginglabeling/labelingnutrition/ucm511646.pdf.

New Label/What's Different

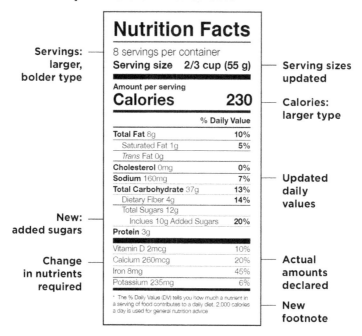

Servings: larger, bolder type

Serving sizes updated

Calories: larger type

Updated daily values

New: added sugars

Change in nutrients required

Actual amounts declared

New footnote

Nutrition Facts

8 servings per container
Serving size   2/3 cup (55 g)

Amount per serving
Calories   230

% Daily Value

Total Fat 8g	**10%**
Saturated Fat 1g	**5%**
Trans Fat 0g	
Cholesterol 0mg	**0%**
Sodium 160mg	**7%**
Total Carbohydrate 37g	**13%**
Dietary Fiber 4g	**14%**
Total Sugars 12g	
Inclues 10g Added Sugars	**20%**
Protein 3g	
Vitamin D 2mcg	10%
Calcium 260mcg	20%
Iron 8mg	45%
Potassium 235mg	6%

* The % Daily Value (DV) tells you how much a nutrient in a serving of food contributes to a daily diet. 2,000 calories a day is used for general nutrition advice

1.   Begin by looking at the number of *servings per package or container* and the *serving size.*

2.   Check out the amount of *calories* per serving.

3.   Check out the *added sugars.* These are sugars added during processing or packaging.

4.   Look at the *% daily values* section. It will help you see how the food fits into your eating pattern. These are the average values for a person eating two thousand calories for the entire day.

5.   Aim for 20 percent or higher for vitamins, minerals, and dietary fiber, and 5 percent or less for saturated fats, trans fats, cholesterol, and sodium.

6. The actual amount is also listed for vitamin D, calcium, iron, and potassium.

Slow Down Aging with Antioxidants

Health experts say antioxidants may help slow aging and fend off age-related wrinkles.[23] Remember, antioxidants are the substances in food that help prevent damage to the cells in your body caused by free radicals, which occur naturally during a process called oxidation. Protecting your cells from damage may protect you from certain diseases. Some important antioxidants in our food include carotene and vitamins A, C, and E.[24]

Vitamin A and Carotene are important for healthy cells, heart, lungs, kidneys, and eyesight. You can get loads of vitamin A and carotene from carrots, tomatoes, collard greens, cantaloupe, broccoli, kale, squash, peaches, apricots, sweet potatoes or yams, and other bright yellow/orange-colored fruits and vegetables.

Vitamin C is necessary to make collagen, which is important to improve your immunity and keep your skin blood vessels, bones, tendons, and ligaments healthy. Vitamin C is found mostly in tomatoes, strawberries, and citrus fruits like oranges, grapefruit, lemons, and limes, as well as in vegetables like spinach, bell peppers,

23 V. Lobo et al., "Free radicals, antioxidants and functional foods: Impact on human health," *Pharmacognosy Reviews* 4, no. 8 (July-December 2010): 118-126, accessed June 1, 2017, on US National Library of Medicine, National Institutes of Health, www.ncbi.nlm.nih.gov/pmc/articles/PMC3249911/.

24   Maeve Cosgrove et al., "Dietary nutrient intakes and skin-aging appearance among middle-aged American women," *The American Journal of Clinical Nutrition* 86, no. 4 (October 2007): 1225-1231, accessed online June 1, 2017, http://ajcn.nutrition.org/content/86/4/1225.long.

and broccoli, and in green leafy vegetables like kale, escarole, collard greens, arugula, and Swiss chard.

Vitamin E is necessary for the proper functioning of many organs in your body. It can reduce and repair damage to the cells in your body and prevent heart disease. It acts as nature's anti-aging vitamin by nourishing your skin and fighting off free radicals that cause wrinkles. Vitamin E is found mostly in nuts and seeds like almonds, hazelnuts, and sunflower seeds, but can also be found in wheat germ and in vegetable and fish liver oils like cod liver oil.

Eat from a Rainbow of Colors with Phytonutrients

It's easy to spot foods rich in phytonutrients in your grocery store because they are usually bright in color. *Phytonutrients* are nutrients found in plant foods, and they pack a lot of punch when it comes to health benefits. They have antioxidant and anti-inflammatory benefits that help improve immunity and may even help prevent certain cancers. Nutrition researchers estimate that there are more than four thousand phytonutrients. A single vegetable like the carrot, for instance, has more than one hundred phytonutrients. Phytonutrients are found in fruits, vegetables, whole grains, legumes, nuts, seeds, and teas. Some herbs and spices—such as turmeric, cloves, ginger, peppermint, and cinnamon—contain plenty of phytonutrients and powerful antioxidants, and are known through history for their medicinal uses.

Phytonutrients are found in fruits, vegetables, whole grains, legumes, nuts, seeds, and teas.

COLOR	PHYTONUTRIENT	HEALTH BENEFITS	FRUIT OR VEGETABLE
Red	Lycopene Anthocyanins Polyphenols	helps control high blood pressure, may protect cells from becoming cancerous strengthens immune function	apples with the skin tomatoes and tomato-based products (tomato sauce, ketchup) beets red cabbage cherries cranberries pink grapefruit red apples red grapes red peppers pomegranates radishes raspberries rhubarb strawberries watermelon
Green	Lutein Indoles	may block cancer-causing substances helps reduce the risk of cancers like breast cancer	asparagus collard greens and other leafy greens kale kiwi green beans broccoli bok choy Brussels sprouts green cabbage green pepper spinach watercress parsley
Yellow/ Orange	Beta-carotene	helps maintain good vision reduces cell damage in the body and improve immunity	apricots butternut squash cantaloupe carrots mangoes nectarines oranges papayas peaches pumpkin sweet potatoes butternut squash
Blue/ Purple	Anthocyanins Flavonoids	creates powerful antioxidants that may help slow the effects of aging helps keep heart healthy helps keep healthy blood pressure, lower risk of cancer, prevent blood clots	blackberries blueberries black currants eggplant purple grapes plums prunes raisins
White	Anthoxanthins Isoflavones	helps lower blood pressure and cholesterol helps prevent inflammation, boost immunity reduces the risk of heart attacks and cancers	chives garlic ginger mushrooms onions leeks scallions

Phytonutrients are found in red/pink foods like tomatoes, guava, and watermelon, blue/purple foods like açaí berries, blueberries, blackberries, and red cabbage, yellow/orange foods like carrots, winter squash, papaya, and sweet potato, as well as green foods like kale, spinach, and collard greens. Some white/creamy colored foods like garlic, onions, and leeks, although not brightly colored, contain phytonutrients and also have many health benefits.

So, eat healthful and dive into a rainbow of phytonutrients;[25] by adding more color to your plate.

Wake Up Your Taste Buds with Juices and Smoothies

If the notion of drinking your vegetables never excited you, now is the time to give it a try. Incorporating fresh fruit and vegetable juices into your diet is a great way to get more phytonutrients and antioxidants. Juicing is a creative way to try fruits and vegetables that you would not normally eat.

There are a variety of power juicers on the market that can extract and separate the liquid and pulp from even the toughest fruit or vegetable. Before you juice, wash the fruits and vegetables with an all-natural fruit and vegetable wash to remove any lingering residue of dirt, bacteria, fertilizer, and pesticides. Some fruits and vegetables like apples, oranges, carrots, and celery naturally contain lots of water, so they will yield more juice. Be creative and juice any combination of fruits and vegetables to get the most nutrients possible. Try a three-to-one vegetable-to-fruit ratio, for example,

---

25   "Phytonutrient rich foods: Add color to your plate," Dana-Farber Cancer Institute, accessed June 1, 2017, https://www.dana-farber.org/uploadedFiles/Library/health-library/nutrition/phytonutrient-rich-foods.pdf.

three vegetables like kale, celery, cucumber to one fruit like an apple.

If there is a downside to juicing, it's that when you extract the juice you are discarding the valuable fiber in the fruits and vegetables. This means you do not get the full benefit of the whole fruits or vegetables. Remember, you need fiber to help monitor your blood sugar and keep your digestive system working. To make up for this, you should eat plenty of whole fruits and vegetables. Remember, you need fiber to keep your digestive system working well.

A word of caution, though, making juice to replace a meal really won't keep you full for very long, and may make you overeat at your next meal. If breakfast in a glass appeals to you, then a smoothie is a substantial option. You can combine whole fruits and vegetables with fresh juice, milk, yogurt, or tofu for your favorite blend.

Give your smoothie more bounce by adding ingredients like almonds, cashews, walnuts, chia seeds, flax seeds, or your favorite protein powder. You will find many juice and smoothie recipes at your fingertips online, and in cookbooks. Experiment and mix and match fruits and vegetables to create combinations to suit your taste.

Create Your Own Juice and Smoothie Combinations

VEGGIES FOR JUICING	FRUITS FOR JUICING	SMOOTHIE ADD-ONS
beets	apples	**nuts**
cabbage	lemons	almonds
carrots	limes	cashews
celery	nectarines	walnuts
collard greens	oranges	**seeds**
cucumber	pineapples	chia seeds
dandelion greens	pomegranates	flax seeds
kale	watermelons	hemp seeds
spinach	tomatoes	pumpkin seeds
spring greens		sesame seeds
swiss chard		sunflower seeds
peppers		**milk/yogurt/other**
wheat grass		**protein**
		almond milk
		coconut milk
		yogurt
		protein powder
		soft tofu

VEGGIES FOR SMOOTHIES	FRUITS FOR SMOOTHIES	HERB ADD-ONS
Veggies from the juicing list above, plus:	Fruits from the juicing list above, plus:	ginger
broccoli	açaí berries	mint
sweet potatoes	avocados	parsley
	bananas	cilantro
	blackberries	
	blueberries	
	cantaloupes	
	figs	
	grapes	
	goji berries	
	guavas	
	honeydew	
	kiwis	
	mangoes	
	papayas	
	peaches	
	pears	
	plums	
	raspberries	
	strawberries	

Chill the fruits and juices to be used.

Juice/Smoothie Recipes

Go Green Refresher

Juice:

- four kale leaves
- one cucumber
- two celery stalks
- one lime, peeled
- one green apple, cored

Makes one to two eight-ounce servings. Approximately 207 calories

Super Duper Strawberry Smoothie

Blend:

- half cup chilled fresh or frozen strawberries
- six ounces plain yogurt
- three ice cubes

Makes one serving. Approximately 190 calories

Papaya-Mango-Kale Fest

Blend:

- one-fourth cup orange juice
- one-fourth cup papaya chunks
- one-fourth cup mango chunks
- one kale leaf

Makes one serving. Approximately 77 calories

Eat Vegetarian

Eating vegetarian is a lifestyle change. If you are thinking about making the switch to a vegetarian diet, you should know what's involved.

- **Lacto-ovo vegetarians** do not eat meat or fish, but include eggs and dairy products like milk, cheese, and yogurt.

- **Lacto vegetarians** do not eat meat, fish, or eggs, but include dairy products.

- **Vegans or strict vegetarians** do not eat meat, fish, eggs, or dairy products. Instead, they eat only plant-based foods.

- **Lacto-ovo-pesco vegetarians** eat fish, chicken, dairy, and eggs. This is a more flexible way to explore a vegetarian diet.

For many people, following a vegetarian diet is credited for halting and even reversing heart disease. One study showed that 89 percent of those on an oil-free, plant-based diet with nutrition counseling had a lower rate of heart disease. Start gradually. First, skip meat or other animal products for a week. Then remove one more each week until you reach your vegetarian diet goals. If you decide to go vegan, eat substitutes you really enjoy. Make sure you include a wide variety of vegetables, sprouts, whole grains (including bran and wheat germ), nuts, seeds, beans, fortified cereals, and fortified soy products (tofu, soy milk) to get enough protein, iron, zinc, B vitamins, and calcium. You can find more great ideas and recipes online and in vegetarian cookbooks.

Balance Calories to Manage Your Weight

Fifty-six-year-old Nicki stared hopelessly into the mirror and realized that her struggle to pull up the zipper on her red A-line dress was pointless. She had always kept a healthy weight and was proud of herself for doing so. But over the past year, she had gone up two dress sizes. "I must have put on a few more pounds over the holidays," she whispered to herself.

It didn't help that her new job as administrative assistant at the university kept her at her desk most of the day. The team in her office took turns bringing in chocolate, candy, and pastries every morning. So there was a steady supply of treats all day long. Unable to resist the constant temptations, she had gained about twenty pounds.

Nicki knew that her 2,500-calories-a-day eating habit and sedentary lifestyle would have to change. At five-foot-seven she weighed 192 pounds and had a body mass index (BMI) of thirty. The BMI is used as a way to determine if one is *overweight* or *obese*. Adults of average height who have a BMI of twenty-five to 29.9 are considered *overweight*, meaning they have too much body weight in relation to their height. A woman like Nicki with a BMI of thirty or above is considered *obese* and generally has a large amount of body fat for her height. In order to lose about one to two pounds a week, Nicki must cut her caloric intake by 500-1,000 calories per day. This would bring her daily intake down to about 1,500-2,000 calories.[26]

Will Nicki be successful in losing one to two pounds a week? Well, that would depend on the other lifestyle and behavior changes she must make.

If you are like Nicki and trying to control your weight,

> **Think of how great you will feel when you are making good food choices and living a more active and healthy lifestyle.**

26 "Finding a balance," Centers for Disease Control and Prevention, accessed June 1, 2017, www.cdc.gov/healthyweight/calories.

you must develop a healthy eating style and increase your physical activity. That means making wise food decisions, cutting back on empty calories in certain foods and beverages, engaging in some form of exercise, and cutting back on the amount of time you spend in sedentary activities that burn few calories. Staying active burns calories that would otherwise be stored as fat. It's a simple equation: "calories out" must be more than "calories in."

Think of how great you will feel when you are making good food choices and living a more active and healthy lifestyle.

Be Healthy—Every Day

Ten Tips for Better Eating

Maintaining a healthy weight takes effort and vigilance. These ten tips will help you better manage your eating habits.

1. **Choose foods low in calories**. Eat the right amount of calories for your age, gender, height, weight, and physical activity. Choose healthy foods and beverages from these food groups—fruits, vegetables, grains, proteins, and dairy—to get the nutrients you need. A registered dietitian-nutritionist can help you determine what you need.

2. **Manage the portions you eat**. Eat only when you're hungry and stop before you feel full. Choose small serving sizes to limit how much you eat.

3. **Reshape your plate**. Eat your meal on a smaller plate. This will keep your portions small because a smaller plate holds less food.

4. **Eat mindfully**. Your mind and body work together when you eat. If your mind is preoccupied while you eat, your brain is

less likely to get the signals that warn you when you're full. Turn off your TV and mobile devices while you eat.

5. **Slow down**. Eat slowly. Pay attention to the tastes, smells, and textures of the food. You are more likely to enjoy what you eat, and you're likely to eat less because you feel full quicker.

6. **Don't deprive yourself**. If you skip meals, you may be tempted to overindulge and eat more later. Eat small portions during the day to keep you feeling full longer.

7. **Eat early**. When you eat dinner before seven o'clock, you are likely to still be active, burning off some calories. When you eat late, the opposite happens. Your metabolism has already slowed down and the food is not used for energy but is instead turned into fat.

8. **Spring clean your eating habits**. Clean out your refrigerator and pantry and get rid of unhealthy foods that sabotage your diet. Stock up on healthy items.

9. **Fill half your plate with fruits and vegetables,** one quarter with whole grains, and the remaining quarter with protein. Include fat-free or low-fat (1 percent) milk and water to complete the picture. Remember, three-quarters of your plate should have plant-based foods on it.

10. **Keep healthy snacks handy**. Keep healthy snacks like grapes, apples, pears, berries, cherries, oranges, carrots, celery, raisins, and nuts portioned and packed in sandwich bags and ready to go. They are lightweight and easy to carry around.

chapter six takeaway

Healthy aging involves making deposits toward your health for longer-term gains. The healthier you are, the more fabulous you are. Slow down aging and stave off diseases by practicing healthy eating—reshape your plate, balance your calories, and eat more whole foods. Keeping a food journal will give you a good idea of your eating habits and help you see what you need to change.

An Exercise for Embracing Your Best Self

Revamp Your Diet

List four new fruits/vegetables you will add to your diet in the coming weeks.

1. _____

2. _____

3. _____

4. _____

chapter seven

Exercise—A "Good Thing"

The New York City Marathon is one of the most exciting and most-watched events in the city. The annual 26.2-mile run starts in Staten Island, winds its way through the five boroughs, and then ends in Manhattan. It is the largest marathon in the world, with over fifty thousand runners finishing the race.

One chilly Sunday morning in November, I joined the crowds lining the route as the runners took to the streets. I found a good spot on First Avenue, where I leaned over the barricades to get a good view as the runners made their way down the street. It was remarkable to see each runner hitting their own stride—some sprinting, some jogging, others walking briskly or merely walking at their own pace.

When I finally decided to leave the sidelines to return home, I found myself picking up speed and running. As I ran, a woman shouted out to me, "Practicing for next year?" I laughed and replied,

"It feels good to run." It confirms that simply being around people engaged in physical activity is motivating.

While regular exercise is crucial for these runners preparing for a marathon, the same is true for women as they age. Exercise can lower your risk for certain diseases and ultimately extend your life. In fact, health experts say a lack of physical activity may be the cause of decline in a person's physical health.[27] Frankly, exercising is one more way to do something good for yourself. Your body will respond to exercise no matter your age, so it's never too late to get fit.

Exercise increases your levels of endorphins and serotonin. These "feel good" neurotransmitters can make you feel upbeat and help you think clearer. In fact, studies show that exercise can boost your brainpower and help lift you out of a depressive state.[28]

Just Move

Does the very thought of exercising turn you off? Look at it this way—exercise is simply a way to *move*. Doing physical activities that encourage you to move more is easier than you think. Although these days some fitness centers offer affordable memberships, the truth is you don't have to join one. Find an activity you like—walking, cycling, jogging, swimming, dancing, or playing a sport. There are plenty of things you can do to build activity into your daily routine.

An important point to remember is to start and end your workout with stretches. Include muscle and bone strengthening activities. Muscle strengthening activities make muscles do work

---

27   Larry J. Durstine et al., "Chronic disease and the link to physical activity," *Journal of Sport and Health Science* 2, no. 1(March 2013): 3-11, accessed June 1, 2017, on ScienceDirect, http://www.sciencedirect.com/science/article/pii/ S2095254612000701#gr1.

28   Ibid.

that they are not accustomed to, and bone strengthening activities produce a force on the bones that help them become stronger. Research shows that strength-training exercises can combat a number of physiologic and functional declines that come with age, like loss of muscle mass and strength. If done regularly two to three days a week, weight training can build muscle strength and muscle mass and preserve bone density, independence, and vitality with age.[29]

Six Ideas to Help You Move:

Start walking. If you're new to a regular exercise routine or just getting back into one, a good way to move again is to walk. One of my favorite activities is walking my dog, Bacardi. When Bacardi trots and picks up speed, I am forced to run with him. When he slows down, I walk. Walking Bacardi comes naturally, so walking will be natural for you, too. You don't need to time yourself, or count steps. Simply start with a normal stride, then pick up the pace as you feel more comfortable. Walking is a lifestyle habit you can adopt for keeps. Take a walk after a meal. Start with fifteen-minute walks and build to thirty minutes. Split the time up by doing two or three ten-minute walks during the day. You may find it easier to build a routine if you walk first thing in the morning before other commitments crop up, or at the end of the day. Before you know it, walking will be a regular part of your daily routine.

Break up your exercise time. If your schedule makes it hard to plan regular exercise, start moving in other ways. Begin inserting some type of activity into your day, especially if you have a sedentary job or lifestyle. Health experts say just ten minutes of cardio exercise three

---

29   R. Sequin and M.E. Nelson, "The benefits of strength training for older adults," supplement, *American Journal of Preventive Medicine* 25, no. 3 S2 (October 2003): 141-149.

times a day can give you a host of benefits. Something as simple as doing jumping jacks, stretches, or leg lifts during TV commercials gets you on the right track.

Be creative. If you feel you are too busy to exercise, you can still fuel your fitness with everyday activities. Get off the elevator one floor before your destination, then walk up the other flight. If you take the bus, get off one stop sooner and walk the rest of the way. If you are driving, park your car farther from your destination and walk the rest of the way. Look for activities in your community. Most communities have dedicated parks and recreation departments that offer a variety of physical activity programs to encourage people to use the local facilities.

Find ways to move indoors. If the weather or allergies prevent you from exercising outdoors, then exercise indoors. Your local shopping mall may let people in early before the stores open, so they can walk laps around the inside perimeter. Gyms, health clubs, fitness centers, and studios also offer classes in dance, Zumba, Pilates, water workouts, tai chi, yoga, and other combination exercises. If price is a factor, there are countless exercise videos on YouTube and on cable TV channels devoted to exercise and fitness.

Exercise with friends or a workout buddy. Add years to your life and work out with someone. One research study found that people over age seventy-five who were physically active and who joined in social activities lived longer than their less social, less active counterparts.[30] When you plan regular walks with a fitness friend, you

---

30 "Staying active and social prolongs life even after 75," Tufts University Health and Nutrition Letter, December 2012, accessed June 1, 2017, www.nutritionletter.

have something to look forward to. These planned activities keep you motivated. You're both more likely to stick to your routine when you have someone to hold you accountable. If you decide to join a fitness center, they may offer free sessions when you bring a workout buddy.

Have Fun with It

Whatever form your fitness program takes, make it fun. Don't think of it as one more thing to do. Think if it as "me time"—time that you have set aside for yourself.

If you haven't exercised for a while, don't overdo it. Start small and go slowly. Gradually build up the intensity and the amount of time you commit to it each day. This way you will avoid workout exhaustion and burnout. If you're like me and have a dog, upgrade your routine from the walks around the block to runs in the park. You will find others doing the same thing.

If you exercise outdoors, keep it stimulating and change where you go. Take your mind off working out by listening to music or watching TV, shifting your thoughts to something pleasant like your last family vacation. You are more likely to keep it up if you don't think of your fitness routine as a chore.

If you "fall off the wagon," get back on it as soon as possible. Don't let a lapse in your routine bring everything to a permanent halt. If you miss a day or two, get back on track and start moving again—that's the only way to make exercise a regular part of your lifestyle.

tufts.edu/issues/8_12/current-articles/Staying-Active-and-Social-Prolongs-Life-Even-After-75_936-1.html.

Get Inspired

Fuel Your Life with Yoga

Last summer, thousands of yoga lovers converged on Times Square in New York, transforming it into a yogi's paradise. As they hit their mats, stretching and balancing in unison, it was enough to inspire the passive onlooker to take up yoga.

These days, more people are taking up yoga than ever before. So, whether you are you are trying to reconnect with your inner self or seeking healing vibrations, you can do yoga almost anywhere—indoors or out, at home, in the park, or on the beach. The quiet, precise movements and poses of this ancient practice require balance and concentration. Health experts attest that yoga can help improve your overall fitness, muscle strength, flexibility, endurance, and body image. In fact, research shows that a single bout of yoga can significantly increase your body image. Yoga can even lower your heart rate and help to manage chronic conditions like blood pressure, cancer, pain, depression, anxiety, insomnia, and fatigue.[31] A beginner's class is the best way to learn and get started. You will be on your way once you get the hang of things.

Start your yoga routine by first finding a tranquil space without outside distractions. If you are indoors, yoga music and gently scented aromatherapy candles can help set the mood. The goal is to get the most out of your routines, not strain yourself. Do stretches and poses only as you feel comfortable. With practice and a good yoga instructor you will become more flexible and be able to do more complex routines later on.

---

31 Harvard Medical School, "Yoga—Benefits beyond the mat," February 2015, accessed November 11, 2016, http://www.health.harvard.edu/staying-healthy/ yoga-benefits-beyond-the-mat. "This workout will make you feel better about your body after one session," www.womenshealthmag.com. June 2016, accessed September 21, 2017.

Yoga Poses for Your Daily Routine

Downward Facing Dog

This pose works your upper and lower body, including your hands, arms, shoulders, back, calves, and feet. It is the *home* yoga position. Whenever I do this pose, Bacardi always jumps in and does the same pose, only he does it better! Makes sense, since he is a dog. It's quite hilarious to see us both on the mat.

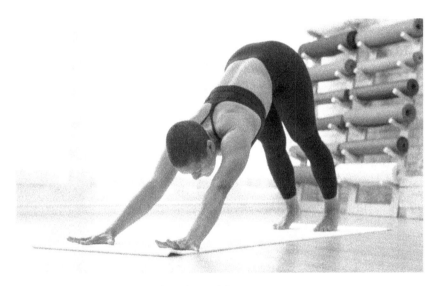

1. Start on your hands and knees.

2. Keep your neck in line with your spine, wrists in line with your shoulders, and knees in line with your hips. Keep your gaze toward the floor.

3. Put your weight on your hands, spreading your fingers wide, with your middle fingers facing forward. Press firmly into the ground using your palms and fingers.

4. Relax your upper back and lift your knees off the floor, bring your toes to face forward.

5. Keep your arms straight but not locked and your spine straight as you lift your tailbone up.

6. Move your chest closer to your thighs to form the shape of the letter A.

7. Your legs may be straight, or you can keep them slightly bent if that makes you feel more comfortable. You should feel a stretch in the back of your legs. Press the heels of your feet into the floor.

8. Breathe, holding this position for four to eight breaths.

9. Release this position, exhaling while you gently bend your knees and lower your hips back toward the floor and return to your hands and knees.

Child's Pose

This pose creates a good stretch in your hips, thighs, ankles, and back.

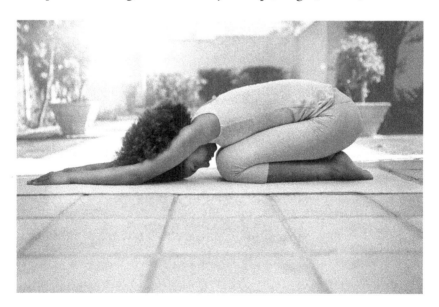

1. Start on your hands and knees with the tops of your feet flat on the floor and your big toes touching each other.

2. With your knees together or spread apart (whichever is most comfortable), gently lower your hips and rest your buttocks on the heels of your feet.

3. Keep your back straight and feel the stretch in your spine.

4. Exhale and move your torso to where it is resting on or between your thighs. Bring your forehead to rest on the floor.

5. Stretch your arms forward with your elbows next to your ears and your palms on the floor. If it feels more comfortable, bring your arms to rest by your sides with your palms facing upward.

6. Relax your elbows, arms, back, and shoulders.

7. Breathe slowly and deeply, keeping your torso on your thighs as you inhale.

8. Hold this position for four to twelve breaths.

9. Release this pose, gently using your hands to walk your torso back to the upright position.

10. Sit back on your heels or place your palms on the floor beneath your shoulders and slowly lift yourself back up to a seated position.

Mountain Pose

This pose creates an invigorating stretch for your arms and torso while improving posture and balance. It is a great pose to do at the start of your day.

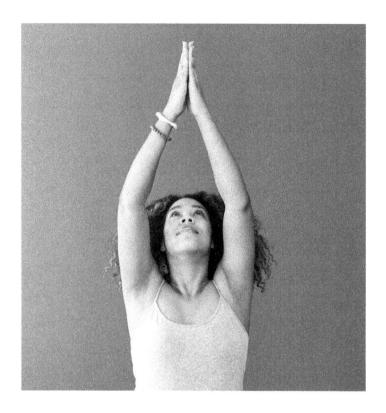

1. Start with your feet hip width apart and parallel to each other.

2. Press your feet into the mat or ground, spreading your toes.

3. Keep your shoulders down, and reach your arms straight overhead as you take a deep breath.

4. Focus on your breath; inhale, then exhale.

5. Release, lowering your arms.

Exercises for Balance and Strength

Remember that it's best to talk with your doctor or health professional before you start any exercise routine. Before you begin these or any exercises, do a short warm up to avoid potential injury to your muscles. A warm up can include five minutes of walking in place, walking outdoors, on a treadmill, or on a stair stepper.

Improve Your Balance

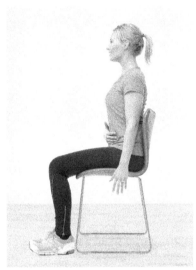

For these next two seated balance and coordination exercises, you will need a sturdy chair that won't slide.

Seated Leg Lifts

This exercise focuses on your lower abdominals.

1. Sit upright in the chair, keeping your back straight.

2. Lift one leg with your knee bent at ninety degrees.

3. Hold your leg up with your foot about six to ten inches off the floor for five seconds.

4. Repeat ten times, then switch to the other leg and repeat the steps.

Seated March

This exercise stretches your hamstrings while strengthening your hips.

1. Sit upright in the chair, keeping your back straight.

2. March your feet up and down twenty times—left, right, left, right, and so on, lifting your feet a few inches off the floor.

Improve Your Strength

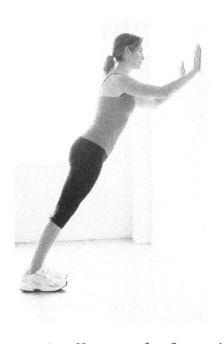

Wall Push-Ups

This exercise is much easier than a floor push-up yet will still strengthen your arms, chest, and shoulders. Use a wall that is free of objects and where the floor is not slippery. Breathe normally during these strength exercises.

1. Face the wall, standing about an arm's length away, and keep your feet about shoulder-width apart.

2. Keep your feet flat on the floor. Lean your body forward and place your palms flat against the wall at shoulder-height and shoulder-width apart.

3. Slowly breathe in as you bend your elbows and bring your upper body toward the wall in a slow motion.

4. Hold the position for one second.

5. Breathe out and slowly push yourself back until your arms are straight.

6. Repeat ten to fifteen times.

7. Rest, then repeat ten to fifteen more times.

Back Leg Raise

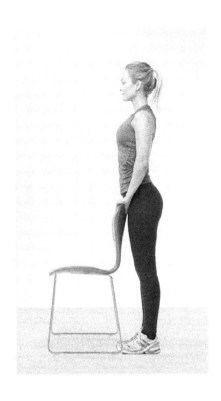

For this exercise, you will need a sturdy chair that won't slide. This exercise strengthens your buttocks and lower back.

1. Stand behind a sturdy chair, holding on for balance. Breathe in slowly.

2. Breathe out and slowly lift one leg straight back without bending your knee or pointing your toes. Try not to lean forward. The leg you are standing on should be slightly bent.

3. Hold position for one second.

4. Breathe in as you slowly lower your leg.

5. Repeat ten to fifteen times.

6. Repeat ten to fifteen times with your other leg.

7. Repeat ten to fifteen more times with each leg.

Side Leg Raise

This exercise strengthens your hips, thighs, and buttocks.

1. Stand behind a sturdy chair with feet slightly apart, holding on for balance. Breathe in slowly.

2. Breathe out and slowly lift one of your legs out to the side. Keep your back straight and your toes facing forward. The leg you are standing on should be slightly bent.

3. Hold position for one second.

4. Breathe in as you slowly lower your leg.

5. Repeat ten to fifteen times.

6. Repeat ten to fifteen times with your other leg.

7. Repeat ten to fifteen more times with each leg.

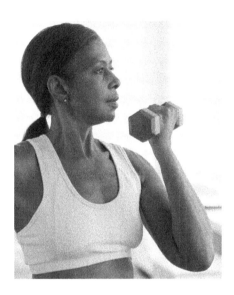

Arm Curl

This exercise can strengthen and tone your upper arm muscles. Start with a five-pound weight (less, if necessary). As you feel yourself getting stronger, use heavier weights and alternate arms until you can lift the weight comfortably.

1. Stand with your feet shoulder-width apart.

2. Hold weights straight down at your sides, palms facing forward. Breathe in slowly.

3. Breathe out as you slowly bend your elbows and lift weights toward your chest. Keep elbows at your sides.

4. Hold the position for one second.

5. Breathe in as you slowly lower your arms.

6. Repeat ten to fifteen times.

7. Rest, then repeat ten to fifteen more times.

chapter seven takeaway

Exercising will increase your "feel good" hormones and give your physical and mental health a boost. Exercise sets the tone for a healthy lifestyle. Start with simple activities like walking, then build up to more intense routines. Make exercise fun, break up your routine, and do it with friends. Include yoga or strength and balance exercises daily.

An Exercise to Embrace Your Best Self

Make Healthy Movement a Daily Habit

1. Get up early and take a sunrise walk. Take a walk after dinner.

2. At least do routines—yoga, or strength or balance exercises daily.

Remember, before you start an exercise program, check with your doctor. Ask if there are any specific activities that you should avoid based on your physical health.

For More Information

"Basic exercise guide for older seniors and the infirm," Peak Fitness, September 11, 2015, http://fitness.mercola.com/sites/fitness/archive/2015/09/11/seniors-basic-exercise-guide.aspx.

"Education," Yoga Outlet, https://www.yogaoutlet.com/guides/.

"Exercise and physical activity: Your everyday guide from the National Institute on Aging," National Institute on Aging, accessed

March 3, 2017, https://www.nia.nih.gov/health/publication/exercise-physical-activity/.

Papa, E.V., X. Dong, and M. Hassan, "Skeletal muscle function deficits in the elderly: Current perspectives on resistance training." *Journal of Nature and Science* 3, no. 1 (2017): 272.

Seguin, R. et al., "Growing stronger: Strength training for older adults," John Hancock Center for Physical Activity and Nutrition at the Friedman School of Nutrition Science and Policy at Tufts University, Division of Nutrition and Physical Activity at the Centers for Disease Control and Prevention, accessed June 1, 2017, http://growingstronger.nutrition.tufts.edu/growing_stronger.pdf.

Wilson, D. et al., "Frailty and sarcopenia: The potential role of an aged immune system," *Aging Research Reviews* 36, (February 2017): 1-10.

chapter eight

Health—Take Good Care of Yourself

Mama put it nicely when she said, "A stitch in time, saves nine." What she meant was, don't procrastinate—take care of a problem before it gets worse. This was not the case with fifty-four-year-old housewife Linda. She had just finished dinner and was watching her favorite TV game show around 8:30 p.m. when she felt a burning sensation in her chest. Thinking that it was only heartburn from the spicy noodles she had just eaten, she dismissed it, took some antacid, and went to bed. But the pain got worse, so Linda decided to play it safe and headed for the emergency room. After an electrocardiogram (EKG) and blood tests, she got the good news that it was not a heart attack after all. She had acid reflux, a condition where the stomach acid moves up into the esophagus (the tube that connects the throat with the stomach). But Linda was not out of the woods yet.

When the doctor read her test results, he discovered some troubling signs. Linda's blood sugar, blood pressure, and cholesterol were out of control. She was a smoker and admitted that she enjoyed drinking most days. She was fifty pounds over her ideal weight for a five-foot-three woman. Her family history was even more worrisome—both of her parents had suffered heart attacks.

Linda was at a high risk for the same fate. Her doctor immediately placed her on medication to control her blood sugar, blood pressure, and cholesterol, and warned her to stay away from cigarettes and alcohol. He referred Linda to a registered dietitian-nutritionist who created a personalized diet and exercise plan for her to follow.

Unlike many women, Linda was one of the lucky ones—fortunately, her first warning was not a heart attack. The truth is, heart disease is no longer a man's disease; it is now the leading cause of death for women in the United States.[32] Linda took the early signals seriously and had enough time to get the proper treatment and avoid a catastrophic outcome.

Embracing good health is not just about discussing and addressing aches and pains. It's about enjoying the best quality of life possible. Enjoying the best quality of life means looking after your own health first. In chapter 4, I mentioned how you must take care of your own well-being before you can be there for anyone else. Think of it as something you would do in an airplane emergency, where you have to put on your own oxygen mask before you can help others.

---

32 "Health equity: Leading causes of death in females," Centers for Disease Control and Prevention, accessed June 2, 2017, https://www.cdc.gov/women/lcod/.

Of course, the more you take care of yourself, the better you will feel—physically, mentally, and spiritually. I see many middle-aged women who are the picture of good health. They look like they take the time to care for themselves—eating right, exercising, having regular medical and dental checkups—even if they have busy lives. Be one of those women. In the process, you will inspire other women to do the same, and take the best care of themselves, too.

Visit Your Health professional

By now, visiting your health professional on a regular basis should be a habit. Choose a provider with the expertise that is a good match for your age and medical needs—someone who makes you feel at ease and who readily addresses your concerns. Whether it's a long-standing family doctor or someone who specializes in women's health issues, you need to forge a good relationship with your health professional. This builds mutual trust and increases your chances of better health outcomes if a medical problem arises.

Today, the patient's bill of rights in hospitals gives patients some control over medical decisions being made. It gives patients the right to ask for copies of their medical records, refuse certain treatments, or even switch health professionals. Gone are the days when patients just nodded their heads to whatever the doctor said. And yet, this is exactly what I used to do. I would leave the doctor's office with lots of unanswered questions. Over the years, I've learned that since I am in charge of my own health, I am ultimately responsible for my own health care. If, for example, the doctor did not explain a plan of care to me, I now know that I have the right to ask questions, and that my privacy will be respected.

In fact, health professionals take notice when patients are fully involved in aspects of their care. With so much information available online, it has become commonplace for patients to ask questions to clear up medical myths and misconceptions.

Make the most of the limited time you have with your health professional by being prepared for your visit. Before your visit, be ready to ask questions about the reason for your visit. Make a list of things you are concerned about. Be specific about any symptoms or side effects of your treatment. Make a list of all the medications and supplements you are taking, including their correct names and the dosages. Some medications may not work well if they are taken together, so it is important that you tell your health professional exactly what you are taking. If tests are prescribed, ask what they are for. Ask how long the treatment is expected to last and ask about the side effects and alternative treatments. Most of all, ask what you need to do to prevent a repeat of your health issue.

Get Your Shots

Talk with your doctor or health professional about which vaccines you need.

The **flu vaccine** is for protection against the influenza virus, which can cause fever, chills, sore throat, stuffy nose, headache, and muscle aches.

The **pneumococcal disease vaccine** is for protection against a serious infection that often causes pneumonia in the lungs, and can affect other parts of the body.

The **shingles vaccine** is for protection against shingles caused by the same virus as chicken pox. If you had chicken pox, the virus still remains in your body. It could become active again and cause shingles.

The **measles, mumps, and rubella vaccine** is for protection against the viruses that cause several flu-like symptoms that may lead to serious long-term health problems.[33]

Get Screened

Getting regular health screenings can help you detect diseases early and prevent health problems in the future. It is a good idea to have regular checkups that include blood tests even if you don't have any symptoms to report. Some health conditions don't always readily show symptoms. High blood pressure, for instance, is known as the "silent killer" and is problematic because the symptoms may not occur until it is very high. There are a number of specific screenings and tests that you should get when you are approaching fifty or are over fifty, but testing things like blood sugar, iron, triglycerides, and cholesterol levels should be routine.

Cervical cancer screening: Women aged thirty to sixty-five should be screened annually, except those who have had their noncancerous cervix removed through a hysterectomy.[34]

---

33 "Age page: Shots for safety," National Institute on Aging, April 2016. https://www.nia.nih.gov/sites/default/files/shots-for-safety_2.pdf.

34 "Prevention guidelines for women 50-64," Johns Hopkins Medicine, accessed June 2, 2017, http://www.hopkinsmedicine.org/healthlibrary/prevention/women_age,50_64/.

Thyroid (TSH) test: This test looks for thyroid disease by measuring the amount of thyroid-stimulating hormone (TSH) your body makes. Women sixty and older should have a TSH test every year.[35]

Mammogram: Women should start having mammograms to screen for breast cancer in their forties and continue every one to two years, depending on their risk factors (like genetics, age, and obesity).[36]

Bone density test: This test tells if you have or are at risk for osteoporosis. These scans should begin at age sixty for women who have an increased risk for fractures and/or have a low body weight. Otherwise the tests should begin around age sixty-five.[37]

Depression: Your emotional health is as important as your physical health. If you have anxiety or depression that lasts more than two weeks, discuss screening and treatment options with your health professional.[38]

---

35   Mary Shomon, "Routine health screenings: What tests should you be getting?" Verywell, April 26, 2016, accessed June 2, 2017, https://www.verywell.com/health-tests-you-should-get-regularly-3232905.
36   "What are the risk factors for breast cancer?" Centers for Disease Control and Prevention, accessed June 2, 2017, https://www.cdc.gov/cancer/breast/basic_info/risk_factors.htm.
37   "Health screening—women—ages 40 to 64," MedlinePlus, accessed June 2, 2017, https://medlineplus.gov/ency/article/007467.htm.
38   "Prevention guidelines for women 50-64," Johns Hopkins Medicine, accessed June 2, 2017, http://www.hopkinsmedicine.org/healthlibrary/prevention/women_age,50_64/.

Your Guide to Screenings and Tests

SCREENING TESTS	AGES 40–49	AGES 50–64	AGES 65 AND OLDER
Blood pressure test	Get tested at least every two years if you have normal blood pressure (lower than 120/80). Get tested once a year if you have blood pressure between 120/80 and 139/89. Discuss treatment with your health professional if you have blood pressure of 140/90 or higher.	Get tested at least every two years if you have normal blood pressure (lower than 120/80). Get tested once a year if you have blood pressure between 120/80 and 139/89. Discuss treatment with your health professional if you have blood pressure of 140/90 or higher.	Get tested at least every two years if you have normal blood pressure (lower than 120/80). Get tested once a year if you have blood pressure between 120/80 and 139/89. Discuss treatment with your health professional if you have blood pressure of 140/90 or higher.
Bone mineral density test (osteoporosis screening)	Discuss your risk for osteoporosis with your health professional.	Discuss with your health professional.	Get tested at least once at age sixty-five or older. Discuss with your health professional.
Breast cancer screening (mammogram)	Discuss with your health professional.	Get tested at age fifty and every two years thereafter.	Get tested every two years through age seventy-four. Age seventy-five and older, discuss with your health professional.
Cervical cancer screening (Pap test)	Get a Pap test and human papillomavirus (HPV) test together every five years.	Get a Pap test and HPV test together every three years.	Discuss with your health professional.
Cholesterol test	Get a cholesterol test regularly if you are at increased risk for heart disease. Discuss your risk factors with your health professional.	Get a cholesterol test regularly if you are at increased risk for heart disease. Discuss with your health professional.	Get a cholesterol test regularly if you are at increased risk for heart disease. Discuss with your health professional.
Colorectal cancer screening (using fecal occult blood testing, sigmoidoscopy, or colonoscopy)	Discuss with your health professional.	Starting at age fifty, get screened for colorectal cancer. Discuss with your health professional.	Get screened for colorectal cancer through age seventy-five. Discuss with your health professional.
Diabetes screening	Get screened for diabetes if your blood pressure is higher than 135/80 or if you take medicine for high blood pressure.	Get screened for diabetes if your blood pressure is higher than 135/80 or if you take medicine for high blood pressure.	Get screened for diabetes if your blood pressure is higher than 135/80 or if you take medicine for high blood pressure.

Manage Stress

Someone once told me that that the word "stressed" is actually "desserts" if you spell it backwards. That's funny when you think about it. Stress can send us craving and seeking comfort in desserts and sweet treats.

On a more serious note, stress is the mental or emotional strain from demanding or frustrating situations. Stress is any situation which tends to disturb normalcy in your body.

Your body responds to *stressors* like tense situations, bad news, being overworked, and issues with family, health, and finances. When you have more stress, your body releases *cortisol,* the main stress hormone. When you have less stress, cortisol levels return to normal, and so does your heart rate and blood pressure. If the stressors are always present, the hormones stay turned on and wreak havoc on your health. That situation is not at all good for your mind, body, and spirit, because over-activation of stress hormones can cause high blood pressure, lower immunity, depression, anxiety, lower life expectancy, and heart attacks. In short, stress kills.[39]

Feed Your Spirit

A healthy lifestyle may slow the effects of aging, so it must include nurturing your spirit and relieving stress. Finding time to meditate is one way to feed your spirit and melt away stress. A survey of CEOs of Fortune 500 companies found that many of them admitted that they meditate. In chapter 4, we explored meditation exercises you can use to help reduce stress.

---

39 Mayo Clinic Staff, "Chronic stress puts your health at risk," Mayo Clinic, accessed June 2, 2017, http://www.mayoclinic.org/healthy-lifestyle/stress-management/in-depth/stress/art-20046037.

In his book, *Don't Sweat the Small Stuff*, Richard Carlson suggests that even when you have a hectic and stressful life, it's best to remain calm. This reaffirms that too much stress is bad for your mental and physical health.

Frankly, stress doesn't have to be a big part of your life. One way I used to de-stress was to tend my garden, pulling up weeds and watering the plants. There is something very thera-

A survey of CEOs of Fortune 500 companies found that many of them admitted that they meditate.

peutic about leisurely spraying water on growing things. So, while gardening might appear to be mindless, successful gardening is much more than reaping flowers and vegetables. For me, it was a form of therapy—it fed my spirit and melted away my stress.

chapter eight takeaway

Good health isn't always associated with illness—it's not merely the absence of disease or physical weakness. Getting screened regularly will detect many health problems before they surface. A healthy lifestyle includes nurturing your spirit and reducing everyday stressors. Make time to meditate.

An Exercise to Embrace Your Best Self

Thirty-Two Ways to De-Stress

Practice at least five of these thirty-two ways to de-stress daily.

1. **Write it down**. Make a list, then prioritize. Do first things first. This prepares you for the day ahead, so you are more proactive and less reactive.

2. **Pamper yourself.** Splurge with a relaxing full body massage, or escape with a luxurious bubble bath and scented aromatherapy candles while you listen to soothing music.

3. **Let go of the past**. Free yourself and forgive yourself and others of past mistakes. When you are wrong, admit it.

4. **Take a break**. Stretch, walk, run, or dance for a few minutes each day. It will perk you up and lift your spirits.

5. **Drink more green tea and eat more super foods**. Eat more blueberries, almonds, walnuts, kale, dark chocolate, flaxseed, chia seeds, açaí berries, and wild salmon.

6. **Go the extra mile**. Take the stairs instead of the elevator, or take a brisk walk outdoors. Breathe deeply and increase blood flow to your body.

7. **Skip the nightly news**. Most of the time, it's not *good* news anyway.

8. **Munch on fruits or veggies**. If you like to snack, apples, pears, peaches, plums, nectarines, oranges, nectarines, grapes, berries, and baby carrots can be little bites of heaven.

9. **Become a micro gardener**. Start an aromatic herb garden in your yard or on your windowsill. Lavender, mint, basil, chives, sage, rosemary, and thyme are easy to grow. The aroma will delight your senses—and add zest to your cooking.

10. **Beat the blues**. Get things off your chest and talk to someone—a professional, a friend, or a family member.

11. **Live in the moment**. Savor joyful moments and even the small pleasures you experience.

12. **Get enough sleep**. Stay mentally alert, and repair and replenish by getting at least seven hours of sleep a day.[40] Go to bed thirty minutes earlier than your usual bedtime.

13. **Indulge in a quiet retreat.** Leave the busy world behind, tune out, and soothe your mind with absolute peace.

14. **Read something inspirational.** Escape from everyday worries and read. You will amp up your brainpower and be mentally stimulated.

---

40 "How much sleep is enough?" National Heart, Lung, and Blood Institute, US Department of Health and Human Services, accessed June 2, 2017, https://www. nhlbi.nih.gov/health/health-topics/topics/sdd/howmuch.

15. **Give someone a helping hand**. The more you help someone, the more it becomes a gratifying habit. You will feel good doing it.

16. **Practice deep breathing.** It recharges your battery, relaxes your muscles, and releases your endorphins—those "happy hormones" that put you in a good mood.

17. **Smile and laugh more**. Smiling is contagious. Laughter is good medicine. Find humor in everyday things and you will be more fun to be around.

18. **Give more praise**. Every day, give at least three people a genuine compliment, something they will feel good about.

19. **Choose to be happy**. Surround yourself with happy people and live each day as if it's your last day to be happy.

20. **Try a fresh look**. Wear a new piece of jewelry or a scarf. Both are always trendy and can make your outfit look brand new.

21. **See a show**. Get tickets for a show you always wanted to see.

22. **Learn something new**. Take an adult continuing-education class, take up a sport, learn to play the piano, paint, or sign up for a dance class.

23. **Start a walking group**. All you need is at least one other person to add to the fun and fresh air. It will make you want to get up and go.

24. **Have an attitude of gratitude**. Start a gratitude journal. Begin or end your day with things you are grateful for. Start each day by thanking your *Creator* that you are alive. You will feel more optimistic.

25. **Look to the skies.** Take time to look up at the sky—the changing shades of blues, grays, and oranges, the clouds and how they float by. Take deep breaths and relax.

26. **Stretch away stress**. If you feel tension in your neck and shoulders, unwind with a few simple stretches or yoga poses.

27. **Keep a cool head**. Stay calm when you are under pressure. You will think more clearly and solve the problem quicker.

28. **Take a "mental health day" off from work**. Get in a few extra *Z*s and bounce back refreshed and revitalized.

29. **Get away alone or with friends**. Explore or just hang loose. You will build great memories.

30. **Unplug from technology**. Disconnect your smartphone, tablet, and other electronic devices now and then. You will clear your head from mental overload and constant stimulation.

31. **Visualize it**. Find a quiet, comfortable spot, close your eyes, and imagine yourself in a place you love, someplace that's healing and comforting, doing something you enjoy. If it's walking on the beach—dig your toes into the sand, feel the warmth of the sun, hear the surf, inhale the clean fresh air.

32. **Listen to music**. Turn on your favorite light music—slow down your pulse and lower your stress hormones.

part three

Your Best Spirit

chapter nine

Be Mindful—Give
Thanks for the Rain

I love being in a classroom, and I love to read and write, but there are times when I'd rather be out in nature than anywhere else. There were days as a doctoral student when I needed to hunker down in the library, but I much preferred being outdoors repotting a plant than at a computer.

I simply got more pleasure out of being with nature, more gratification from its pleasurable diversions.

Some women have trouble taking time to enjoy the simple things around them. Appreciating the simple things take mindfulness, a focus or awareness on the present. It is emotional intelligence and the ability to look within but still be present in the world around them. A calm acknowledgment or acceptance of your body's sensations and feelings in a given moment will set the tone for how you begin to care for your spirit.

Care for Your Spirit

The World Health Organization defines health as "a state of complete physical, mental, and social well-being."[41] I would suggest adding "spiritual well-being" to complete this definition. That's the definition that should ring true for women at any age.

In today's fascinating high-tech world, the vast majority of us don't take the time to savor precious moments in life. We tend to spend much of our time busy with "life"—work, home, TV, and mobile devices. As a result, we miss out on the natural beauty the world offers and on having good old-fashioned fun.

Now that you've reached an age where you can slow down and appreciate life more, it's time to look for ways to find balance and care for your spirit. One way to do that is to connect with nature.

Connect with Nature

In nature, things are surviving, growing, thriving, and evolving. Looking out my window in late fall, I can see that the leaves have disappeared from the trees. I know they will return again in all their splendor when spring arrives. Like nature, you must grow and evolve. But mostly, you want to thrive, not just survive—and that takes nurturing. You need nurturing to stay alive and healthy. Just as you tend a garden to keep it green and growing, you must tend your spirit in order to grow and thrive.

This nurturing can come from spending time connecting and being in harmony with nature. There's so much magnificence in nature. Think about how we share the park with the wildlife—bees buzzing from flower to flower collecting nectar, boastful butterflies

---

41   "About WHO," The World Health Organization, who.int, http://www.who.int/about/mission/en/.

dancing from leaf to leaf, birds tweeting to their mates or eagerly pecking at seeds. Then there are the flowers—how do those amazing roses manage to fold their petals so neatly? How does a peony in its lush fullness hold up those heavy blooms after they burst into marvelous, plush balls of colors? What are those tiny wildflowers that appear out of nowhere called?

Exploring and enjoying nature can be fascinating and good for you.

Exploring and enjoying nature can be fascinating and good for you. Many parks have nature trails that make it easy to explore, watch birds, or learn about the plants and creatures that make the park their home.

So care for your spirit by spending time in nature this week, and let its sights, sounds, and scents fill you. Soak up a little sun, feel the breeze against your face.

Bring the outdoors in with a potted plant or herb. Lavender, mint, basil, rosemary, and thyme are not only beautiful and easy to grow, but they also bring healing aromatic scents to your space.

If not herbs, then color your world with flowering plants. One study found that women living with green vegetation around their homes lived longer than those who didn't.[42]

If you have an office, add some foliage to your workspace with flowering plants—with care, most will last a long time. My friend, Caitlin gave me an orchid plant as a gift, and after the flowers were gone, it stayed alive and healthy for more than a year.

42 "Women Live Longer in Areas with More Green Vegetation," National Institute of Environmental Health Sciences, https://www.niehs.nih.gov/research/supported/sep/2016/women-live-longer/index.cfm

Terrariums or a simple cactus can also add greenery. Bring fresh-cut flowers home once a week; you will find that most markets carry inexpensive bunches of fresh cut flowers year round. A tabletop water feature can also bring in sounds of a soothing waterfall to your space. There are even mini zen gardens made up of sand and pebbles that can bring a bit of the outdoors in.

Nature has its own healing power. Connecting with it is a wonderful way to help you keep your spirit serene yet upbeat. It can boost your creativity, slow your pulse, lower your cortisol levels (stress hormones), create spontaneous happiness, and ultimately enrich your life.

Nurture Your Relationships

Caring for your spirit also means connecting and fostering mutual bonds of friendship with people who make you feel optimistic, positive, and cheerful. I discussed the value of making those connections in chapter 2. The old saying, "The more the merrier," makes sense; a Gallup poll found that, "When people had almost no social time in a given day, they had an equal chance of having a good day or a bad day. However, each hour of social time quickly decreased the odds of them having a bad day. Even three hours of social time reduced their chances of having a bad day to 10 percent."[43]

For the sake of your mental and social well-being, it's time to make the time to nurture your community of friends. It doesn't take much to nurture friendships with people who bring rays of sunshine into your world. My friend Trish knows this. She often sends e-cards, and they always seem to come at the perfect time. Her last card read:

---

43   Tom Rath and Jim Harter, "Your friends and your social wellbeing," Business Journal, August 19, 2010, accessed June 2, 2017, http://www.gallup.com/businessjournal/127043/friends-social-wellbeing.aspx.

"Thinking of you. Sending hearts, hugs, butterflies, and warm positive energy your way." So send a cheerful "Hello" card, or call, email, text, FaceTime, or use other forms of social media to connect with a friend. Make "It's Just Coffee," or "Sip and Say," dates. You'll be investing in your social circle and nurturing your spirit at the same time.

Take the Time to Enjoy Music

In college, I studied classical and neoclassical music and learned to appreciate the music of composers like Stravinsky, Bach, Verdi, Beethoven, and Mozart. I developed an ear for different movements of musical compositions, and the contributions of each instrument in an orchestra. Today, I still listen for different instruments in a musical arrangement, regardless of the genre. For instance, when I hear a song by Earth, Wind & Fire—one of my favorite musical groups—I have a deep appreciation for the depth of the musical arrangement. I hear the horns and the percussion and understand how many layers compose the melody of the song.

There's also something therapeutic and healing when you listen to music. Music therapy is a well-established health profession that is used to treat physical, emotional, cognitive, or social conditions. It is used in conventional medicine, and in integrative and alternative medicine practices, as a nonmedical approach to health and healing.[44] Listening to relaxing music before surgery can make people less anxious. Some doctors play music while they perform in-office procedures, dentists play music as they drill, and people listen to music to make their exercise easy or to ease pain and tension. So, not only can listening to music give you a deeper appreciation for talent, but it is also undeni-

---

44 "Music therapy," The Ohio State University Wexner Medical Center, accessed June 2, 2017, https://wexnermedical.osu.edu/integrative-complementary-medicine/music-therapy.

ably a form of therapy for your spirit. If you've not tried it, listen to music for entertainment, and listen to it for your health.

Start a Gratitude Journal

When you appreciate the things around you, you are developing "an attitude of gratitude." I've mentioned having this attitude in previous chapters; now let me explain how to cultivate it. Research shows that cultivating an attitude of gratitude results in better psychological and physical health. One study showed that people who were more grateful were more optimistic about life, and had fewer visits to the doctor than those who focused on aggravation.[45]

Start each morning with a positive note. In anticipation of the day ahead, write seven to ten upcoming things or events for which you are grateful.

A great way to develop an attitude of gratitude is to start a "gratitude journal." Get a journal or notebook, or use an app on your mobile device. Start each morning with a positive note. In anticipation of the day ahead, write seven to ten upcoming things or events for which you are grateful. At the end of the day, journal again, this time reflecting on any seven to ten things that happened over the course of the day for which you are grateful.

Keep it simple. You don't have to be grateful for just the big things; be grateful for the small things, too. Be grateful for people, opportunities, situations, experiences. Be grateful that you received a compliment,

---

45 "In Praise of Gratitude," Harvard Health Publishing, health.harvard.edu, (November 2011): https://www.health.harvard.edu/newsletter_article/in-praise-of-gratitude.

completed a project on time, or felt the warmth of the sun or the gentle summer rain that cooled things down on a hot day. Of course, you should be grateful if you received a raise, your cholesterol results came back normal, or you purchased a new condo at a steal.

Other things to be grateful for:

- something you were worried about worked out well

- making a new friend

- professional milestones or goals achieved

- successes of a friend or family member

- finding something you lost

Your gratitude journal is a great tool for shifting your mindset from negative to positive. Focusing on the positive helps to uplift your spirits. You'll create a certain aura that is bound to attract positive energy into your life. You might be amazed at the good things that begin to happen once you start having an attitude of gratitude.

Declutter Your Life

Have you ever said to yourself, "I can't go to sleep," "I can't create," "I can't concentrate," "I'm not thinking clearly," or "I need to clear my head"? Then you probably have too many things cluttering your mind—and your space.

Clutter isn't just having too much *stuff* stacked in a disorganized fashion around you; your mind can also have too much clutter. An example of mind clutter might be worrying about things you can't control. You may be cluttering your mind with things that are irrelevant. The emotional impact of clutter reinforces distress; it causes you to be agitated and unable to think clearly amid all the stuff.[46]

So far, I have discussed meditation, breathing, journaling, and yoga as things that can, in essence, help you mentally declutter. Your efforts to maintain your best mental health can be more effective when you also declutter your space—your house, your car, your closets, your office, your pocketbook. Decluttering will help you redefine who you are at this point in your life.

If you don't have enough room to move around, can't find things you have, and don't know what you really have, it's time to get rid of things you no longer need. Give yourself breathing room and start by clearing out your physical space. There is something freeing about clearing out and creating order in any place you occupy. Consider furniture, clothing, bills, receipts, papers, magazines, equipment, things that loved ones and grown children left behind, and mementoes that no longer have any sentimental value. By clearing out the space where you live, you're creating a vacuum—opening up yourself for a free flow of energy, and for more goodness to enter.

While you are at it, take the time to declutter your relationships, too. Now is the time to decide whether you want to continue to invest in relationships with people who are pessimists or who seem to always have a dim outlook on life. These are the people who criticize others, gossip, and unload hostility. If the time spent in their company isn't uplifting, consider whether you want to continue investing in the relationship, or peacefully detach from them.

Make a list of people who are in your life for your *highest good*—those who bring value to your life. These are the people who make

---

46   Jennifer Baumgartner, "Your closets, your clutter, and your cognitions," Psychology Today, blog, February 29, 2012, accessed June 2, 2017. https://www.psychologytoday.com/blog/the-psychology-dress/201202/ your-closets-your-clutter-and-your-cognitions-1.

you feel comfortable, optimistic, and cheerful when they are around. These are the people who call you up and are upbeat and genuinely interested to hear about how *you* are doing. Of course, you need to be there when your valued friends reach out to you for help. After all, "A friend in need is a friend indeed." In those instances, be a good friend, listen, and give them the support they need.

Once you have decluttered your relationships, remember to make time to keep in touch with those you decided to keep.

Rate Yourself on the Life Wheel

By now you might be asking yourself, "How am I doing?" "Is my plate too full?" "Am I thriving or just surviving?" The Life Wheel exercise can help you answer these questions. It can help you be more mindful of the steps to take to be fabulous and healthy over fifty.

The Life Wheel is a tool that many life coaches use in their practices. It gives clients a snapshot of how they are doing in life. The Life Wheel can help you see how satisfied or fulfilled you are, and shows you if you have balance and well-being in your life.

A Gallup study of people in over 150 countries identified career, social, financial, physical, and community as the five "universal elements of well-being." Not surprisingly, the study pointed out that these five elements make the difference between lives that thrive and lives spent suffering.[47]

The Life Wheel focuses on eight segments that represent areas of life and the levels of satisfaction within each. All eight segments are equally important. Each segment is rated on a scale of zero to ten. Zero means you are not satisfied with that area of your life, and ten

---

47   Tom Rath and Jim Harter, "Your friends and your social wellbeing," Business Journal, August 19, 2010, accessed June 2, 2017, http://www.gallup.com/businessjournal/127043/friends-social-wellbeing.aspx.

means you are really satisfied. An in-between rating, like a five or six, means that there are things you need to work on in that segment.

Life Wheel

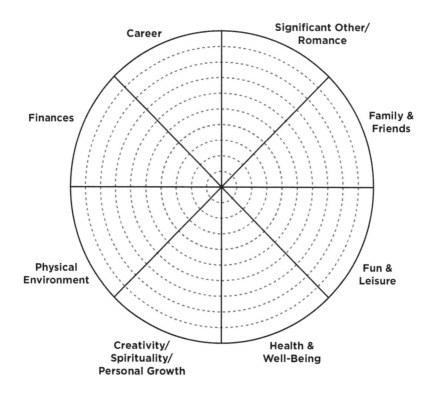

The Eight Elements and What They Mean

Career: If you work, do you like your job? Are you growing and advancing professionally?

Significant other/romance: Do you have love in your life? Do you feel loved? This does not have to be romantic love. If you do not have romance, do you have people in your life who fill that void?

Family and friends: Are you connected to others? Do you have good relationships with your family and friends? Do you talk with them often?

Fun and leisure: Do you have hobbies that you enjoy? Do you take enough time off for rest and relaxation?

Health and well-being: Is your lifestyle healthy? Do you follow a healthy diet? Do you exercise and get enough sleep?

Creativity/spirituality/personal growth: Are you in tune with the universe, your higher self, a higher power, your Creator, God?

Physical environment: Are you living in a comfortable, safe, pleasant, stress-free environment?

Finances: Do you have a good income? How well do you manage your money? Do you save? Do you have any assets? Do you have enough money to do the things you want to do now?

chapter nine takeaway

Giving thanks is good for you mentally and physically. Starting a gratitude journal broadens your perspective about life. Nature provides an atmosphere of tranquility, conducive to contemplation, reflection, and inspiration. Connect with nature and nurture your spirit.

Declutter your environment, mind, and relationships. A personal check-in with yourself can rate your satisfaction with where you are in your life today.

An Exercise for Embracing Your Best Self

Create Balance in Your Life

Complete the Life Wheel and rate yourself according to how satisfied you think you are in each area. Then connect the lines to make an inner wheel and see where you are.

What is the shape of your wheel? Unless you rate yourself a perfect ten in all segments, it should look like a web. The bigger your web, the better you are doing overall. The next step is to reflect on the areas of your wheel where you gave yourself a low rating. Ask yourself these questions:

- In what segments do I have low ratings?

- What am I putting on hold?

- What have I been neglecting?

- What areas do I need to work on right now?

- What changes do I need to make?

- How will I do it?

- How soon will I do it?

Set goals to start working on the areas where you had the lowest rating. For example, if you gave yourself a four for Finances, a goal might be, "Starting next payday, I will arrange for a direct deposit of X into my savings account every two weeks."

chapter ten

Affirmations—Think Positive

One day, a colleague of mine gave me a nice compliment on my hair. "What do you use in your hair?" she asked. "Every time I see you, your hair looks so healthy and shiny. How do you get it to look like that?"

Up to that point, I had never really thought about my hair looking a specific way to other people. I always made sure my hair looked good when I dressed. I often switch things up a bit and wear one of my snazzy lace-front wigs, but I never thought about the specific impression my hair made on someone else. Some of these compliments I receive have become self-affirming.

Using affirmations, or words and phrases, to acknowledge and appreciate simple attributes about yourself or a situation can instill positive thoughts and feelings in your mind and inspire and motivate you.

Something psychological happens when you do self-talk. Sometimes little whispers come into your thoughts, and they're not always positive. This is unlikely to bring you positive inspirations. On the other hand, positive self-talk can make you feel good. That's what affirmations do. They reprogram and retrain your unconscious mind to remove self-limiting beliefs. They rewire your brain and work to create surges of creative energy. They keep your spirit alive and upbeat.

Begin Your Good from the Inside

Experts in the positive-thinking field say, "Thoughts are things." Affirmations, then, are things that help you begin to have your best life experiences and feel good from the inside. When you feel good inside and when you feel good about yourself, it shows. You exude self-confidence and have a certain aura that the world sees. Affirming yourself can help release those "feel good" neurotransmitters— serotonin and endorphins.

On the other hand, when you voice the negative, you're affirming the negative. For instance, if you say you're depressed or in a bad mood today, you're setting the stage for feeling lousy. Voicing the negative can be a self-fulfilling prophecy and potentially attract negativity.

So if you're going to predict something about yourself, why not predict something good? Affirmations are deliberate ways to replace negative thoughts with positive ones in any situation. They can be powerful short sentences, phrases, or statements that you repeat to yourself. They are often soothing and uplifting, and can empower you by helping you find inner peace and cultivate self-love. Think of affirmations as your internal dialogue. They are another way to raise your spirits, improve your attitude about things, and make you feel better about yourself.

More importantly, affirmations are an ideal addition to your morning meditation routine. If you wake up and you feel excited, use that as an affirmation—"I'm feeling excited about today," "I'm happy to be alive," "I'm happy to see a new day." Affirmations can be done any time of the day. Consider using them as part of the mirror exercise that I shared with you in chapter 1,

Affirmations are deliberate ways to replace negative thoughts with positive ones in any situation. They can be powerful short sentences, phrases, or statements that you repeat to yourself.

or as part of your gratitude journaling. Or you can simply repeat them to change the way you view things. Even if saying affirmations feels a bit odd at first, have fun with it and take it in stride—but continue to use them.

That's what Pat—a fifty-three-year-old group leader at a large retail chain—did when she used positive self-talk to turn around her fear of public speaking. Pat dreaded public speaking, and for years she managed to avoid speaking up in meetings at work. Her biggest fear was that she might say the wrong thing. On occasions when she was asked a question, she would get choked up and her voice would quiver when she spoke.

When Pat's boss asked her to give a twenty-minute presentation about creating in-store displays, she panicked. Her fears reinforced her belief that she would say the wrong thing. Then she remembered reading that positive self-talk can help change how people perceive themselves, so she began a daily practice of positive self-talk to bolster her self-confidence. She made a list of uplifting affirmations to repeat to herself:

- I am articulate.

- I am certain that I have something important to say.

- I am able to speak in a clear voice.

- I am eager for people to hear me speak.

- I enjoy speaking to large groups of people.

- I am confident.

- I am more knowledgeable about this subject than my audience.

- I am certain that I've got what it takes to do this.

She repeated the phrases every morning when she woke, while she got dressed, during the day, and before going to bed. When she began shifting her language, she redirected her negative feelings to positive ones.

The positive self-talk paid off. That week, Pat gave the presentation without a hitch, and she has given several presentations since then. These days, she teaches merchandising part-time in an undergraduate college program, and uses positive self-talk often.

Like self-talk, visual affirmations can be very effective in bringing good vibrations to your home or office. Displaying a bit of your inner spirit in your living and working spaces can also inspire others who enter it. For instance, using the concepts from the old Chinese art of *feng shui*, you can arrange your space to alter the flow of energy and bring about positive changes in your life. This creates an inspiring, inviting, and tranquil feel and helps to raise your mental energy.

Natural light, plants, artwork or photos with positive and uplifting messages, a favorite quote, wall ornaments, and tabletop items with affirmational phrases will not only spice up your décor, they can also change the mood. In my office, I have a plaque that says "I am not here to be average, I am here to be awesome," and my favorite mug reads, "Live well, laugh often, love much." So, find those words and phrases that you like and use them.

Change Your Life with Affirmations

In chapter 1 I discussed flipping the script. In order to flip the script, your affirmations should be positive. They should be upbeat and should shift your vocabulary from "I *can't*" to "I *can*."

Whether you choose to do a mirror exercise or write down your affirmations, name positive things you like about yourself.

1. Create positive images as you go—hair is manageable today, your beautiful smile. Don't be surprised if your list gets longer and longer. Whatever you do, don't nitpick over what you view as physical features you dislike.

2. Next, list some things you want in your life—self-confidence, a better work life, home, or business environment, financial independence, future successes.

3. Once you have your list, begin writing out a short statement about each.

4. Keep them specific and positive. Use "I am" (two powerful self-assuring words) instead of "I will." Dreaming big is okay, but be realistic. It's unrealistic to affirm "I am growing taller" if you are short.

5. Keep your affirmations in the present tense—no need to defer them to the future.

6. Repeat them daily, in a confident voice and with conviction, putting your emotions into it when you speak.

chapter ten takeaway

You are fabulous. Love yourself with affirmations. Using affirmations is one way to acknowledge and appreciate your attributes or a situation. Instilling positive thoughts and feelings in your mind will inspire and motivate you. Flip the script and make your self-talk upbeat and positive. Even if saying affirmations feels odd at first, just have fun with it and continue to say them. Begin now to create your own affirmations, starting with things you like about yourself.

An Exercise for Embracing Your Best Self

You Are Special—Love Yourself
Here are other affirmations for you to consider. Of course, personalize your affirmations, using your own words as they apply to you.

- I am beautiful.

- I am born to greatness, with many God-given talents.

- I am articulate.

- I am fun and easy to get along with.

- I am healthy from head to toe.

- I am confident I am abandoning old habits, and practicing good habits.

- I am guided with every step I take.

- I am loving, lovable, and loved.

- I am experiencing happy, healthy relationships.

- I am seeing myself happy in my new home.

Now create a few affirmations of your own.

I am _____

I am _____

I am _____

I am _____

chapter eleven

Embrace the Tough Times

If you've seen the romantic comedy *Moonstruck* starring Cher and Nicholas Cage, you couldn't possibly miss the scene where Cher's character, Loretta, slaps Cage's character, Ronny, and delivers the epic line, "Snap out of it!" A pretty harsh statement if you are experiencing a tough time. "Snapping out of it" is easier said than done. But that's exactly what people sometimes need to do to pick themselves up and get on with life after a difficult situation. Whether it's feeling moody, depressed, or experiencing unresolved grief, at some point they just have to try to "snap out of it."

The fact is, nearly everyone hits a rough patch sometimes—a period where there seems to be a stumbling block or two. Losing a loved one, a health issue, a relationship breakup—these can be particularly difficult. It may be difficult to figure out how to recalibrate, be excited about life again, and start a new chapter.

If this is you, acknowledging the issue you are facing is the first step to resolving it. As I sometimes like to tell people, "When the horse is dead, you must dismount." You have to recognize that it's time to move on, or find something to help you feel good again.

Remember, if you are experiencing concerns that some middle-aged women face—looking older, slowing down, having health, finance, or social issues, or finding yourself with a diminishing number of family and friends—you're not alone.

As I've shared with you in the previous chapters, there are many ways to get around the challenges of growing older. It's up to you to take the first step. Your ability to conquer your challenges is boundless.

For instance, if you find yourself kid-free and alone, consider it liberating. Now you can do some of the things you've put off, some of the things you've always wanted to do. Certainly, events like losing a loved one take time to overcome and heal before you can move on. But when you feel ready, there are several social networks and meet-ups for people over fifty that you can explore.

You may find that after a while you actually enjoy living alone—many women do, and they are alone but not lonely. They are having fun getting out, making new friends, and finding new companionships.

If you're retired or you've chosen not to work full time, consider getting involved in community activities or some kind of humanitarian work. As I mentioned in chapter 2, research shows that volunteers lived longer than non-volunteers when their motive was a desire to help others. Why not volunteer at a local hospital? Seek out an activity that enriches the lives of other people—chances are, you'll find the experience enriching and fulfilling.

Who knows what you can accomplish? Your potential to succeed at new things is limitless. Just look at long-distance swimmer Diana

Nyad, who made history when she swam from Cuba to Key West, Florida. She did this in fifty-three hours at age sixty-four—without the protection of a shark cage. That's a huge accomplishment for anyone, let alone for someone in their sixties. "You are never too old to chase your dreams," Diana told a CNN reporter after swimming the grueling course.[48] It was her fifth attempt after four other tries (one in her twenties and three in her sixties), but she pushed through, and when she arrived in Florida, she told the crowd, "We should never, ever give up. … You are never too old to chase your dreams."[49]

So get ready, harness your energy, pull yourself up by the shoe straps, and start planning and doing things you never had a chance to do. Stay active and focus on restoring your resilience.

When it's called for, bring in the heavy artillery—meditation, yoga, positive thinking, affirmations—to combat situations that threaten your mental health and overall well-being. The heavy artillery in my arsenal is prayer. When some people feel powerless in the face of a trying situation, they often turn to prayer.

> **So get ready, harness your energy, pull yourself up by the shoe straps, and start planning and doing things you never had a chance to do**

---

48   Matt Sloane, Jason Hanna, Dana Ford, "'Never, ever give up:' Diana Nyad completes historic Cuba-to-Florida swim," CNN, September 3, 2013, accessed June 3, 2017, http://www.cnn.com/2013/09/02/world/americas/diana-nyad-cuba-florida-swim/index.html.

49   Ibid.

Use the Heavy Artillery—Pray

Merriam-Webster's defines prayer as, "An address (as a petition) to God or a god in word or thought; an earnest request or wish." The rituals for prayer vary, and it takes different forms—you can say it or think it. At its core, prayer is about communicating from the heart with your *Creator*. It's about renewing your spiritual connection anytime you wish.

Interestingly enough, a poll conducted by the Pew Research Center found that more than half of Americans said they pray every day.[50] But although some people may not admit that they pray, they're probably doing so without realizing it. Every time they say, "Oh my God," or "I pray that you make it home safely," they're praying.

Whether we realize it or not, prayer is everywhere, and people use it every day for many reasons. They pray for reassurance. They pray to be calm. They pray for help to offset negative feelings and situations they encounter. People pray because they want good things to happen to them, or to ask for favors and divine intervention. They pray to be kept safe. They pray to get well from an illness. They pray for forgiveness, and to be able to forgive others. They pray to be nicer to others, and pray for people to be nicer to them. Prayer may even help people build closer relationships, especially when they are in a group that prays together.

In fact, in the medical profession, patients have been shown to make remarkable improvements after praying for better health. That's one reason most hospitals have a chaplaincy department entirely dedicated to meeting the spiritual needs of patients who request it—some patients rely on having a minister, priest, rabbi, imam, or spiritual advisor visit

---

50 "Religious practices and experiences," *US Public Becoming Less Religious*, Pew Research Center, November 3, 2015, accessed June 3, 2017, http://www.pewforum.org/2015/11/03/chapter-2-religious-practices-and-experiences/#private-devotions.

and pray with them. They place a lot of value on being able to communicate with someone and renew their spirit and their spiritual connection with something outside of themselves.

It doesn't take a special language to pray; prayer can be done anytime, anywhere. Growing up, I remember prayer was a more formal exercise—kneeling at the bedside, palms together, then saying a prayer. These days, people utter prayers when they're walking, driving, before they eat, sitting at their desk, in a meeting with business associates, or at a gathering with friends. So take a moment every day to utter a word of prayer, wherever you are—when you wake up, when you're on the road, when you're at work. And while you are at it, remember to give thanks, too.

Use Other Forms of Prayer

In previous chapters, I talked about the benefits of nurturing your spirit through nature. Nature is another piece of heavy artillery to use when times get tough, giving us tools to help us heal from the stresses we encounter and offering gifts that we sometimes miss if we don't get out and explore it. Recently I vacationed with friends, driving though several western states—Utah, Wyoming, and Idaho—and I was amazed at the natural beauty I saw, such as red rocks, and arches formed from years of erosion and geologic activity. And although it was during the height of summer, I could see rows and rows of snow-capped mountains in the distance. The contrast of the rugged terrain and the scenic landscape of the national parks was absolutely breathtaking. So get up, get out, and see some places new in nature. You can retreat into your own world in places like these to quiet your mind and make it a prayerful, meditative experience.

Forgive and Forget

Forgiving someone after you've had a falling out is easier said than done. But holding onto grudges and unresolved hurt can affect more than your emotional health; it can affect your physical health, too. Without forgiveness in your arsenal, your pent-up feelings and emotions can make you harbor anger, anxiety, and resentment. These emotions can cause stress and depression. Studies have found that when you forgive, you reap huge rewards for better health—improved cholesterol levels, better sleep, lower heart attack risk, lower blood pressure levels, and less pain, anxiety, depression, and stress.[51]

Forgiveness is letting yourself off the hook. When you forgive, you are actually doing something good for yourself: you're freeing yourself of bitterness and hostility. Think about the emotional value that you'll have when you "let it all go." Who needs all that extra emotional baggage? So don't hold grudges, move on. Offer empathy and kindness to anyone you feel has wronged you. Writing about your feelings in a letter or a journal, or talking about issues with someone else, will give you peace of mind and emotional relief.

Prayers like the Lord's Prayer or the Prayer of Saint Francis captures it all. I like this prayer as a way of praying not only for myself but also for others and for the world. Regardless of your belief systems, make up a similar tribute of your own. Ask how you can be an instrument for a better world.

Prayer of Saint Francis

Lord, make me an instrument of your peace:
where there is hatred, let me sow love;

---

51 "Forgiveness: Your health depends on it," Johns Hopkins, accessed June 3, 2017, http://www.hopkinsmedicine.org/health/healthy_aging/healthy_connections/ forgiveness-your-health-depends-on-it.

where there is injury, pardon;
where there is doubt, faith;
where there is despair, hope;
where there is darkness, light;
where there is sadness, joy.

O divine Master, grant that I may not so much seek
to be consoled as to console,
to be understood as to understand,
to be loved as to love.
For it is in giving that we receive,
it is in pardoning that we are pardoned,
and it is in dying that we are born to eternal life.
Amen.[52]

---

52 "Peace Prayer of Saint Francis," Loyola Press, accessed June 3, 2017, http://
www.loyolapress.com/our-catholic-faith/prayer/traditional-catholic-prayers/
saints-prayers/peace-prayer-of-saint-francis.

chapter eleven takeaway

When tough times show up, decide when it's time to move on. Whether we realize it or not, prayer is everywhere; people use it as part of their arsenal to improve themselves or situations. The art of forgiveness and letting go is a powerful tool. You have the power and the potential to succeed at any age.

Embrace Your Best Self

When You Need to Pick Yourself Up

Know that there are indeed ways to pick yourself up and get going again for better days.

Thirty Tips for Better Days

1. Embrace your age.

2. Live with the three Ps: *positivity, pride,* and *presence.*

3. Believe in yourself.

4. Love yourself.

5. Give yourself the attention you fully deserve.

6. Send flowers to yourself.

7. Make a personalized health checklist.

8. Keep your doctor appointments.

9. Upgrade your look.

10. Eat wholesome, healthy foods.

11. Take time to do some form of physical activity every day.

12. Look for the good in people and situations.

13. Spend time with people much older than you, and with people much younger than you.

14. Each night before you go to bed, complete the following statement; "I am thankful for _____." "Today my *wins* were_____."

15. Boost your mood and spirit. Avoid negative self-talk. Change your language to positive self-talk.

16. Make time to refuel—meditate, affirm, pray.

17. Watch movies that make you feel good.

18. Live with purpose and intention.

19. Find something you enjoy doing—and do it.

20. Choose the meaning you give to your life experiences. It's your story.

21. Spend less time with people who have "glass half-empty" views.

22. Spend more time with people who have "glass half-full" views.

23. Set aside quiet "me time" for yourself every day.

24. Do something to make a difference somewhere.

25. Celebrate your accomplishments, even the small ones.

26. Beautify your space.

27. Take a five- to ten-minute afternoon power nap.

28. Get good sleep every night.

29. Play a game or read something that stimulates your brain.

30. Enjoy the ride.

An Exercise for Embracing Your Best Self

Starting now, write down four ways you can be an instrument of peace.

1. _____

2. _____

3. _____

4. _____

conclusion

Now's the Time— Embrace Your Best Self and Be Fabulous and Healthy

The Good News!

The Society of Actuaries says a sixty-five-year-old woman actually has a 50/50 chance of living another twenty years.[53] What's more, a Harvard article said that "Today's sixty-five--year-olds are likely to spend nearly two more years of their remaining lives free of disabilities."[54] The CDC also has a better prediction for the life

---

53 "Actuaries Longevity Illustrator," The Society of Actuaries, longevityillustrator.org.

54 Michael Chernew et al., "Understanding the improvement in disability free life expectancy in the U.S. elderly population," NBER Working Paper Series, Scholars at Harvard, June 2016, accessed June 3, 2017, http://scholar.harvard.edu/files/cutler/files/w22306.pdf.

expectancy of women—we are living into our eighties.[55] That is amazing news for all of us women! It means we are not only living longer, but we can expect to be healthy and active without debilitating disabilities.

In the introduction to this book, I mentioned the three Ps: positivity, pride, and presence. Remember, *positivity* is about having an upbeat outlook and a positive essence in your mind, body, and spirit. *Pride* is about being and celebrating your best self, and letting the world see it. *Presence* is about exuding confidence. Combined with the themes, stories, and exercises I've shared, I hope you now have a sense of how these three concepts can play out at this point in your life. Living the three Ps prepares you for your next chapter in life. You believe in yourself and are proud of your accomplishments. You're keeping your brain alert by playing more and doing more. You're taking the time to practice meditation, yoga, tai chi, prayer, affirmation, or something new. You're making more effort to make someone else happy. You are practicing gratitude. You've come a long way, proving that you are indeed a *Life Expert* and a *Life Teacher*, and you willingly share your talents. You know what to do to keep in optimal shape—physically, mentally, and spiritually—for the years to come.

As you begin to develop new relationships—friends, family, and community—new experiences will begin to open up. By now, you are already making great progress. Remember to tap into being around people much older and people much younger than yourself. You will find that you have much to learn from each other. Older people offer you history and a legacy of experiences, they are the storytellers. Younger people help you stay in touch with what's new,

---

55 Jiaquan Xu et al., "Mortality in the United States, 2015," Centers for Disease Control and Prevention, National Center for Health Statistics, December 2016, accessed June 3, 2017, https://www.cdc.gov/nchs/products/databriefs/db267. htm.

showing you new ways of seeing life. They'll make you feel energized to do things that you dared not do before.

Throughout this book, I've explored some of the ways to revitalize your spirit, care for yourself, love yourself, feel fulfillment, and be empowered to age gracefully.

I hope this book will serve as a guide to help you through this most exciting chapter of your life. When you need a good perspective about what makes this time in your life worthwhile, go back and read—and practice—the exercises that I've shared. They will help you find new ways to age gratefully and gracefully, knowing that more good awaits you.

It's time to reclaim your physical and mental health by spring cleaning your eating habits, and being physically and socially active. Remember, vigorous health means you are fiercely resilient and more in control of your life. With the positive ingredients in this book, you have a winning recipe for health, balance, and well-being to embrace your best and be fabulous and healthy after fifty.

Dare to believe in yourself and have confidence in yourself. Create a powerful vision and a clear direction of what's next for you. In the words of Ralph Waldo Emerson, "Once you make a decision, the universe conspires to make it happen."[56]

> **Dare to believe in yourself and have confidence in yourself.**

So stay inspired. As a woman over fifty, you have many unique strengths to harness, and you have intuition and insights to do more great things. Always look on the bright side. It will fuel your passion

---

56 "Ralph Waldo Emerson quotes," BrainyQuote, accessed June 3, 2017, https://www.brainyquote.com/quotes/quotes/r/ralphwaldo383633.html.

to explore ways to age gracefully and get the most out of life. It's true: "Part of the fun is in the journey." Embracing the changes that come with age *will be your greatest journey yet.*

How exciting it is to find new ways to reinvent yourself and enjoy life. Why not make your journey fun and event-filled? Be optimistic as you look ahead, and affirm for yourself that life can be *greater later.*

The best is yet to come. Your next chapter can be your best chapter. *Embrace your best self and be fabulous and healthy beyond fifty!*

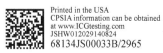
Printed in the USA
CPSIA information can be obtained
at www.ICGtesting.com
JSHW012029140824
68134JS00033B/2965